Living with

Series editors: John Riordan and Bob Whitmore

Each book in this series will deal with a chronic serious disease or condition. It will contain background and medical information on causes and symptoms and will explain treatment in some detail — both practical (drug treatments, surgery) and psychological (self-help, home care, social implications)

already published

Living with stress and anxiety
BOB WHITMORE

**Living with
breast cancer and mastectomy**
NICHOLAS TARRIER

Living with dementia
JOHN RIORDAN and BOB WHITMORE

Living with back pain
HELEN PARKER and CHRIS J. MAIN

Living with stroke
PAUL KING

published with this title

Living with tinnitus
DAVID W. REES and SIMON D. SMITH

Living with
anorexia and bulin

Living with
anorexia and
bulimia

JAMES MOOREY

Manchester University Press

Manchester and New York

Distributed exclusively in the USA and Canada
by St. Martin's Press

Copyright © James Moorey 1991

Published by Manchester University Press
Oxford Road, Manchester M13 9PL, UK
and Room 400, 175 Fifth Avenue,
New York, NY 10010, USA

Distributed exclusively in the USA and Canada
by St. Martin's Press, Inc.,
175 Fifth Avenue, New York, NY 10010, USA

A catalogue record for this book is available from the British Library

Library of Congress cataloging in publication data
Moorey, James. 1954-
    Living with anorexia and bulimia / James Moorey.
        p.   cm. — (Living with)
    Includes bibliographical references (p.   ).
    ISBN 0-7190-3368-3 (hardback).
    1. Anorexia nervosa. 2. Bulimia. 3. Adjustment (Psychology)
I. Title. II. Series.
RC552.A5M66 1991
    616.85'26—dc20   91-19478

ISBN 0 7190 3368 3 *hardback*
ISBN 0 7190 3369 1 *paperback*

Typeset in New Century Schoolbook
by Koinonia, Manchester
Printed in Great Britain
by Bell & Bain Ltd, Glasgow

044931

Contents

In memory of Janet French

Acknowledgements

I would like to thank Debra Stackwood for her typing and editing skills. I would also like to acknowledge and thank all those whom I have worked with in therapy, both those struggling with anorexia or bulimia and their families.

Preface

This book has been written for all those involved in trying to help people with anorexia or bulimia. This includes parents, brothers, sisters, spouses, and friends of sufferers, as well as members of the various 'helping professions', such as GPs, nurses, social workers, occupational therapists, etc. But it is also hoped that this book will be read by sufferers themselves, both for general information about anorexia or bulimia, and for practical suggestions that may help recovery.

The first four chapters answer questions of a factual nature: what are anorexia and bulimia, how are they identified, and what causes these conditions? Chapters 5 to 9 focus on practical issues: how to help, and what kinds of therapy are available. Throughout the book I have made reference to individuals with anorexia and bulimia, and their families, that I have worked with in therapy. In each case their names and certain details have been changed. Although chapters 5 to 8 are aimed at particular groups of people, for example parents in chapter 5, it is hoped that all of these chapters will be read together as the topics dealt with in each chapter are by no means only relevant to the group to which the chapter is primarily addressed.

Throughout this book I have referred to those who fulfil the diagnostic criteria for anorexia or bulimia as 'anorexics' or 'bulimics'. I also use the feminine pronouns 'she' and 'her' when referring to sufferers from these conditions. But it should be borne in mind that diagnostic classification tells us nothing about the unique and varied individuals who receive such labels. Also while the overwhelming majority of sufferers are female, males with anorexia or bulimia are in just as much need of help and attention, and the material in this book will be just as applicable to their needs as to female sufferers.

Parents, relatives and friends of people suffering from anorexia or bulimia often ask: 'How can we help?' They also very often hide the extent of their own suffering. This book has been written in the hope that the information provided here will both offer guidance on how anorexics and bulimics can be helped,

and also assist and encourage families who face the very difficult task of living with anorexia or bulimia.

James Moorey

1 Anorexia and bulimia: what are they?

Anorexia nervosa refers to a condition of self-imposed starvation, characterised by severe weight loss. Bulimia nervosa refers to the habitual eating of large amounts of food (bingeing), followed by purging (usually vomiting), these episodes of bingeing and purging often alternating with periods of self-imposed starvation, but without the sustained weight loss typical of anorexia nervosa. Both involve similar preoccupations with body shape and weight, and an intense desire to be thin. Why should an apparently healthy, normal individual systematically starve themselves? How can we make sense of this behaviour?

These actions seem all the more incomprehensible when we consider how most people react to the prospect of limited food supplies. Starvation has been one of the perennial threats to mankind. From the earliest written records to the present day the devastating effects of famine are clearly documented. Food shortages provoke anxiety and, if the shortages are severe enough, panic and even murder. For example, Josephus, a first-century Jewish historian, describes the siege of Jerusalem by the Romans in AD 70 and recounts how the occupants were driven to extreme lengths to obtain food, finally even to cannibalism as the siege led to severe food shortage and the city's population began to starve.

However, in contrast to these reports there are many accounts of people who have apparently chosen to starve themselves, often to the point of extreme emaciation, in some cases to the point of death. How are we to understand their behaviour? This chapter will examine various forms of self-imposed starvation and the reasons given for this action. This will enable us to compare and contrast these examples with the self-imposed starvation characteristic of anorexia and bulimia and hence be clearer about the various ways of answering the question: what are anorexia and bulimia?

Purification and protest

When someone voluntarily restricts food intake we may say they are 'fasting'. However, we say of someone who has voluntarily reduced their food intake to a point where health is endangered that they are 'starving'. Some medical authorities suggest that after 24 hours of fasting starvation begins. There are many descriptions of people who have starved themselves to a point of extreme emaciation. One such account concerns the experience of Gautama Siddhartha, the Indian prince who founded Buddhism 2,500 years ago. During his search for enlightenment Gautama employed a number of traditional Indian ascetic practices, one of which was fasting. He starved himself to the point where his 'limbs became like knotty sticks and his spine which could be grasped from the front through the flabby skin of his abdomen was like the rough weave of a braid. His protruding thorax was like the ribbed shell of a crab and his emaciated head was like that of a gourd that had been plucked too soon and had withered as a dried up well ... (he) was only skin and bones.'

Gautama had embarked on the course of asceticism as a way of subduing the flesh in order to attain a spiritual goal. The essence of the practice is purification, or the removal of obstacles, on the path of spiritual attainment. The legends tell us he abandoned this path and eventually reached his goal through a 'middle way' of moderation. According to the records he seems to have had no difficulty abandoning the ascetic path once he had decided it would not have the effect he desired. Given the assumptions of the tradition in which Gautama acted, in particular the need to subdue physical appetites, his self-starvation is understandable. However, without that essential information, derived from the context in which he acted, his behaviour would be very difficult to understand. Fasting for religious purposes is a custom with a very ancient history, examples of which can be found in many parts of the world. But again in each case the behaviour becomes comprehensible when we take account of the beliefs and desires of the individual, and the culture in which they act.

The culture of India is also extremely rich in examples of our second type of self-imposed starvation. Whereas the first type concerns efforts motivated by religious aspirations and aims to alter the inner state of the person who fasts (which I have broadly labelled purification), the second form explicitly aims to draw attention to, or change, some external state of affairs. Essentially these are examples of protest. It was common practice in India for a man who wished to collect a debt to fast outside the door of the debtor until the debt was settled. A more familiar example is that of Gandhi who used self-starvation as a powerful political weapon against the British. Of course Gandhi's use of fasting served many purposes: the essentially religious aims of purification and penance as well as the political aims of drawing attention to injustice, protest and attempting to induce change in others. Although in the case of Gandhi we find his fasts motivated by a number of reasons and with various objectives, once again given access to this information his decision to starve himself is comprehensible.

In Europe we can also read many accounts of self-imposed starvation which we may broadly classify as purification or protest, or in some cases a mixture of both. One example is that of St Wilgefortis (the name literally means 'strong virgin'), who was the daughter of a Portuguese king of the 10th century AD. Wilgefortis starved herself rather than marry the Saracen King of Sicily 'in order to preserve her virginity'. When the Sicilian King saw how emaciated Wilgefortis had become he broke off the marriage engagement. The Portuguese King was so enraged at his daughter's behaviour that he had her crucified. After her death she was hailed as a martyr and became the focus of various cults throughout Europe. A British psychiatrist, J. Hubert Lacey, has suggested various features of this account may lead us to conclude that Wilgefortis was actually what we would recognise as anorexic. He suggests that while this could not be regarded as the first written description of anorexia nervosa, it may be the first account which indicates the psychological foundations of the disorder. This view has been challenged and it is difficult to assess this example clearly as so much myth has been woven into the accounts. However, the behaviour of Wilgefortis may be explained as both a protest against an arranged marriage, and an expression of her desire to dedicate her life to God.

There are a great many examples of self-starvation among women in the late and post-medieval periods in Europe. These women, termed 'Holy Anorexics' by Rudolph Bell in his book on the subject, embarked on a course of extreme asceticism in the context of a Christian culture considerably less inclined towards such practices than it had been in earlier centuries. These women were often regarded as saints by local communities. At first appearance we seem to be considering examples of self-starvation motivated by a specifically religious quest for self-purification. However some writers have presented a case for regarding the ascetic practices of these women as being essentially acts of protest, or even revolt, one aspect of this rebellion being the rejection of a conventional arranged marriage through disrupting their own sexual responses and reproductive capacity by means of self-starvation. This act of defiance against parental and social pressures occurred in the context of an increasing secularism, materialism, and tendency to religious moderation. As such it may have served as a profound rejection of the new values which had been embraced by their families. Caroline Bynam has drawn attention to the way in which the asceticism of the women served not only to defy the family and social pressures to accept an arranged marriage, but also served to carve out a specifically female identity in a religious structure dominated by male power. These examples may therefore be seen as attempts to exert power on the part of people in a situation where they are apparently without power. Hence, it is argued, the meaning of self-starvation in these instances revolves around issues of power and identity, not simply religious aspiration. Once again we should note that the social context, beliefs, and desires of the people concerned provide us with explanations of what would otherwise be incomprehensible behaviour. Although we need to recognise that in these examples the objectives may not have been explicit, that is their motivations may have been, in some sense, 'unconscious'.

In Europe the use of self-starvation for explicit political ends can be seen with the suffragettes, who went on hunger strike in protest at imprisonment. It is interesting to note that prior to the suffragette movement examples of the explicit use of self-starvation as a political weapon were almost exclusively used by men, while examples of female self-starvation are most often seen in a religious context, as noted above. Many other examples of the use of the 'hunger strike' as a method of protest, or to bring political pressure, may be cited: for example, in recent years in Northern Ireland. In the case of the politically motivated fasting (the hunger strike) we usually see an attempt to influence the course of events by people denied access to other methods of producing political change. The important point to note here is that these incidents can only be understood when we examine the social and political context, the beliefs and desires, of the people involved.

Fraud and exhibition

The above section has looked at the role of self-starvation in the context of political or religious aspiration, examples of which can be noted throughout recorded history. But we also have a number of accounts of self-imposed starvation that do not have an identifiable religious or political motivation. Some of these became notorious as examples of fraud. One example is that of Sarah Jacob ('The Welsh Fasting Girl'). Over a period of 26 months from October 1867 to November 1869 Sarah and her family claimed she had eaten nothing. This period of alleged total abstinence from food had followed a period of reduced food intake and weight loss which began when Sarah became ill in February 1867. Although she appeared to recover and began to eat in March 1867 she gradually reduced her food until stopping completely in October. The case of this 'miraculous faster' received a great deal of publicity and Sarah received many visitors who would often leave money. Contemporary accounts do not describe Sarah as emaciated, in fact she appeared well despite being thin. Eventually a local committee of medical and professional men organised a vigil to observe Sarah so they could check the claims that she was surviving without food. After 18 days Sarah became ill and died. Although the parents were punished with imprisonment it seems likely that it was Sarah who had deceived her parents and ate secretly over the 26 months of the alleged fast. A number of writers have drawn attention to some interesting features of this type of account. Supporters of these women tended to talk in terms of their 'miraculous' ability to survive without food, while those wanting to investigate the likelihood of fraud were usually highly suspicious and hostile, hence incidents of fasting girls often became a focus for religious versus scientific attitudes. Certainly these women attracted much attention and some, in addition to notoriety, acquired money. Even in those accounts of women who were found to be frauds, we can often detect, in addition to considerable hostility on the part of investigators, an equally deep fascination.

In the nineteenth and early twentieth centuries a great deal of interest was aroused by 'hunger artists', or 'exhibition fasters', people who voluntarily starved themselves and were exhibited in public. These people were essentially professional fasters. Periods of total abstinence from food ranged from 20 to 50 days during which members of the public could pay to come and observe their condition. Self-starvation as a public spectacle occurred in the context of the Victorian obsession with oddities and 'the miraculous'. Again it has been suggested that this obsession was a reaction to the growth of the scientific world view which was threatening to debunk many long cherished religious and supernatural beliefs. Whatever the motivation, people flocked to see emaciated men and women who seemed to provide a popular display of the unusual that met public needs at the time. Again we should note that many of these accounts of self-starvation have been explained in terms of the individual's desire for financial reward, or even notoriety.

Health and beauty

The use of fasting to improve health and beauty has been practised in many parts of the world for thousands of years. Sometimes fasts of considerable length were recommended. Avicenna, the great Arab physician, routinely prescribed fasts of three weeks or more. As well as improving physical health, fasting has been employed to improve psychological functioning. For example, in Ancient Greece, Socrates, Plato and Pythagoras all employed prolonged periods of fasting to help them attain greater intellectual clarity. Today, approaches to health care such as 'Nature Cure', and the 'Natural Hygiene' movement, recommend fasting for a wide range of health problems, and even to improve appearance, through cleansing the skin and hair. Again, given the desire to be healthy and certain beliefs about the value of fasting in health care, even extended periods of food abstinence may be comprehensible.

It is possible to identify a range of motivations for self-induced starvation. We can read accounts of people starving themselves for religious, political, even financial reasons. These reasons may not always be regarded as satisfactory explanations for the behaviour but we need to note that self-starvation can be a rational act. But can any of the types of situation discussed above include cases we would recognise as anorexia nervosa? The next section describes the first clinical accounts of anorexia nervosa from the seventeenth century. Before this we have noted some writers consider examples of the condition can be found in the Middle Ages and even earlier (e.g. St Wilgefortis in the 10th century). However, the information on these people is insufficient to allow unambiguous identification of the condition. Some theorists who have looked at the socio-cultural origins of anorexia nervosa have argued that the condition occurred very rarely if at all in the Middle Ages because society was so different at that time. Others disagree and claim that it is likely that there were examples, which are perhaps less obvious because they occur in the midst of socially accepted forms of self-starvation such as fasting for religious purposes. Among the women supposedly exposed as frauds (remember the claim usually involved eating nothing) and the 'Hunger Artists' it is more likely that some were suffering from anorexia nervosa. The next section considers the identification of anorexia nervosa as a medical problem.

'A peculiar form of disease'

From the seventeenth century we have descriptions of people who have starved themselves in circumstances which, it is claimed, are very unlike those we have discussed so far. Here we are not dealing with forms of religious activity or protest, or any other behaviour comprehensible in terms of a person's beliefs and desires. Rather, we are dealing with an illness. In 1689 the English physician Thomas Morton described two cases of what he called 'consumption of nervous origin'. The two patients he described were a young woman of 18 years and a young man of 16 years. Concerning the young woman he wrote: 'Mr Duke's Daughter, in St Mary-Axe, in the year 1864, in the eighteenth year of her age ... fell into a total suppression of her Monthly Courses from a multitude of Cares and Passions of her Mind.

From which time her Appetite began to abate ... She wholly neglected the care of herself for two full years, till at last being brought to the last degree of Marasmus ... and thereupon subject to frequent Fainting Fits, and apply'd herself to me for Advice. I do not remember that I ever did in all my practice see one that was conversant with the Living so much wasted ... (like a Skeleton only clad with skin).'

Morton describes what would be recognised today as characteristics of anorexia nervosa: severe weight loss, cessation of menstruation, particular psychological disturbance, and absence of illness which could explain weight loss (see next chapter for details of diagnosis). Morton was careful to distinguish this condition from consumption (i.e. tuberculosis), and attributes the condition to mental or psychological causes. As weight loss can accompany many forms of illness the identification of a 'wasting' disease which may be distinguished from all other known illnesses was a crucial step.

A form of self-induced starvation has been identified which is not rendered comprehensible through the categories of religious aspiration, political endeavour or protest, deception or exhibition, at least not at first glance. If we want to think about this condition we must do so in different terms: specifically the category of an illness associated with psychological disturbance (a disease 'of nervous origin'). Morton's work is the first clearly identifiable step in the medical understanding of anorexia nervosa.

Although several accounts of what appear to be anorexia nervosa were published in the seventeenth century it was not until the second half of the eighteenth century that the condition received systematic attention. The term 'anorexia nervosa' (which means 'loss of appetite of nervous origin') was first used by the eminent English physician William Gull in 1874. Six years previously, in an address at Oxford, Gull had described 'a peculiar form of disease' which involved severe weight loss, refusal to eat, loss of appetite, amenorrhoea (i.e. loss of menstruation), alertness and lack of lethargy (the latter characteristic allowing differentiation from tuberculosis). He noted the condition usually occurred in young women and named it 'apepsia hysterica'. In his 1874 paper Gull introduced the term 'anorexia nervosa' because there was no absence of the digestive enzyme pepsin and, unlike hysteria, the condition could occur in males. Gull noted his patients were mainly between the ages of 16 and 23, and described two cases in some detail, both of which were female, one aged 17 and one 18. Like Morton nearly 200 years previously, Gull believed the illness to be of psychological origin. He wrote: 'The want of appetite is, I believe, due to a morbid mental state ... that mental states may destroy appetites is notorious, and it will be admitted that young women at the ages named are specially obnoxious (i.e. liable) to mental perversity.'

In 1873 the French physician Ernest Lasègue published a report on a condition he termed 'anorexie hysterica'. His account was based on eight women aged between 18 and 32. Once again the condition is carefully differentiated from other illnesses which may cause weight loss, although Lasègue argued the condition was a form of hysteria. Lasègue was careful to emphasise the mental state of his patients, he wrote: 'What dominates in the mental condition of the hysterical patient is, above all, the state of quietude – I might almost say a condition of contentment truly pathological. Not only does she not sigh for recovery, but she is not ill-pleased with her condition, not withstanding all the unpleasantness attended with.'

The work of Gull in England and Lasègue in France mark the starting point for the modern study of anorexia nervosa. In the century following these initial reports anorexia nervosa has been the subject of considerable controversy. Medical and psychiatric opinion, while consistently regarding the condition as an 'illness', has found it extremely difficult to specify what sort of illness it is. Is anorexia nervosa a physical illness or a mental illness? For most of the last century anorexia nervosa has been regarded as a form of mental illness. However, from about 1914 up to the late 1940s it was widely believed that the weight loss associated with anorexia nervosa was caused by a disorder of the pituitary, a small gland at the base of the brain that plays a crucial role in the regulation of the body's hormonal system. Hence, during this period anorexia nervosa was regarded as a physical illness. It was only after a considerable amount of research, and argument, that the view of anorexia nervosa as an illness of psychological origin with weight loss being attributed to self-imposed starvation, was finally re-established.

Although anorexia nervosa has been regarded as an illness of psychological origin (or a 'mental illness') for the greater part of the century or so since the work of Gull and Lasègue, it has proved extremely difficult to say what sort of psychological disturbance it is. One of the major distinctions made by psychiatrists is between psychotic and neurotic conditions. Briefly stated a psychosis is a mental disturbance which involves delusions or hallucinations. A neurosis is a disturbance of mood, thinking, or behaviour, which though it may be seriously disruptive, even incapacitating, does not involve delusions or hallucinations. In addition to these two broad categories psychiatrists recognise and treat a range of other problems, for example various forms of addiction, such as alcoholism. In trying to answer the question, 'What is anorexia nervosa', medical research has had to consider whether anorexia is a form of psychosis or neurosis, or a form of mental illness distinct from psychotic and neurotic conditions. Another problem has been to establish whether anorexia nervosa is a 'distinct clinical entity'; that is, does the condition exist in its own right as an independent illness, or is it a variation of some other illness?

The history of the attempts to classify anorexia nervosa is very complex. Anorexia nervosa has been regarded as a neurotic condition (for example as a form of hysteria, or a form of obsessive-compulsive disorder), and as a psychotic condition (for example associated with schizophrenia or manic depression). Some have argued the condition lies between the two categories, being 'psycho-neurotic', or 'pre-psychotic'. It is no exaggeration to say that anorexia nervosa has been identified with all the major categories of psychotic and neurotic conditions, as well as many other conditions outside of those categories. It has also been argued that anorexia is a form of malingering. Others have argued that it does not exist as a distinct condition, but is always secondary to some other major disturbance such as hysteria, phobias, compulsive states, depression, psychopathy, etc.

A major problem with the classification of anorexia nervosa has been that loss of appetite may occur in a wide range of psychiatric conditions, and anorexia nervosa itself may involve various psychological symptoms. Hence the very real difficulty of separating anorexia nervosa from other conditions with similar features. In 1963 British psychiatrist A. King published a paper in which he suggested distinguishing 'primary' from 'secondary' anorexia nervosa. He argued the former involves notable consistencies in symptoms and personality, with the central feature being a desire to avoid food in order to lose weight, while the latter presents with variable symptoms and fears centering on the process of eating itself.

Most prominent workers in this field have accepted King's position, but there are numerous attempts to define 'primary' anorexia nervosa. Professor Arthur Crisp, whose work has been extremely influential in this field, considers primary anorexia nervosa to be a 'weight phobia', specifically centering on a fear of pubertal weight. He suggests starvation becomes a means of avoiding the adjustment demands of puberty and involves a unique form of regression: 'anorexia nervosa is a defensive biologically regressed posture pivoting around the events of puberty'. Gerald Russell similarly regards the condition to be essentially a 'morbid fear of being fat'.

Recently a number of writers have suggested anorexia nervosa is best regarded as a form of addiction, either to the effects of starvation, or to the sense of control severe food restriction involves. For example G. Szmukler and D. Tantam in a paper published in 1984 compare anorexia nervosa with alcohol dependence and note significant similarities between the two conditions. They suggest viewing anorexia as a 'dependence disorder', rather than a neurosis or a psychosis. Specifically they consider anorexia to be most appropriately regarded as an 'addiction to starvation'.

Some writers still consider anorexia nervosa to be a physical illness, claiming the weight loss and psychological changes are the result of a physical abnormality. It is argued that the fact that in about 20% of cases amenorrhoea occurs before appreciable weight loss, is evidence that there is a prior physical dysfunction. The main hypothesis is that the symptoms of anorexia nervosa result from an injury to, or disease of, part of the fore-brain known as the hypothalamus, which plays a crucial part in regulating body temperature, body weight, appetite, sexual behaviour, blood pressure, and fluid balance. However evidence has shown that hypothalamic disorder in anorexia nervosa is related to degree of weight loss. Also, once weight is restored to levels approximating that expected for the individual's sex, age, and height, symptoms of hypothalamic dysfunction are reversed. These facts suggest that anorexia nervosa is not a product of a diseased hypothalamus. Hence, although research continues into the possibility of a purely physical cause for anorexia nervosa, the position remains a minority view.

In a paper in 1979 Gerald Russell discussed what he called 'an ominous variant of anorexia nervosa', a condition he termed 'bulimia nervosa'. Bulimia refers to a pattern of eating large amounts of food in a short time (bingeing) followed by purging, usually vomiting. This often alternates with periods of starvation. The term ('la boulimie'), had been used in French medical and psychiatric literature since the eighteenth century, and a cycle of bingeing and vomiting had been described in advanced stages of anorexia nervosa. However, from the 1970s accounts of women apparently locked into the binge-purge cycle, sharing similar preoccupations with weight and body shape but without the weight loss characteristic of anorexia nervosa, began to appear. Various terms for the condition have been proposed. Boskind-Lodahl termed the condition 'bulimarexia', in what appears to be the first paper on the subject which was published in 1976. Other terms for the condition include 'binge-purge syndrome', and 'dietary chaos syndrome'. In view of the central feature being a similar preoccupation and anxiety surrounding body shape and weight it has been argued that bulimia nervosa is a subgroup, or variant, of anorexia nervosa, although the relationship between anorexia and bulimia remains an area of dispute.

We have noted in this section that over the last 100 years there has been considerable controversy within medicine regarding the classification and understanding of anorexia nervosa. However, most medical authorities would now agree that primary anorexia nervosa is a form of mental illness, a distinct clinical entity, with at least one subgroup (bulimia), and that the characteristic clinical picture (weight loss, amenorrhoea, etc.) is a consequence of self-imposed starvation.

Starvation as symbol and metaphor

To claim that anorexia and bulimia are symbols, or metaphors, is to claim that they represent or stand for something. That is, they have a specific meaning. There are a number of variations of this view but the essential claim is that in some way anorexia and bulimia represent, or express, the position of women in our society. Some of those who would regard anorexia and bulimia in this way would accept that they are rightly considered as illnesses, but point out that they are illnesses with a special meaning for our time. Susan Sontag, in her book *Illness as Metaphor*, discusses tuberculosis in nineteenth century Europe and notes that the condition, while of course remaining a terminal illness, became a symbol, or a metaphor, for a romantic, sensitive, enlightened, refined, but tragic, higher nature. In a sense it became fashionable to have tuberculosis, and the condition came to stand for, or represent, certain values. But of course tuberculosis was nonetheless a disease. The life style which led some to develop the condition may well have been an expression of choice or even protest, but this did not alter the status of tuberculosis as a physical illness.

Now some would insist that although it may be true that a person may become physically ill through severe emaciation or recurrent bingeing and vomiting, it is incorrect to regard the decisions and actions that lead to these problems as themselves symptoms of illness. It is claimed that people do not 'get' anorexia and bulimia, as we would get tuberculosis, influenza, or cancer. Rather anorexia and bulimia are 'modes of being', or ways of coping; they are life styles, or stances, not diseases. This view would reject the language of medicine as inappropriate to a discussion of the nature of anorexia and bulimia. Anorexia and bulimia are seen as political choices, or statements, intimately connected with our society's view of, and treatment of, women.

Although there may be disagreements about whether anorexia and bulimia should be considered illnesses, the cluster of views which see them as ultimately political, are an important strand of current thinking on eating disorders. American psychologist Richard Gordon in his book on the socio-cultural roots of anorexia and bulimia notes: 'The politics of eating disorders ultimately revolve around the politics of gender. The contemporary epidemic of these conditions is a reflection of the ambiguities of female identity in a period of change and confusion.' The problem of establishing a coherent sense of self, of female identity, in a culture saturated with contradictory demands on women, is a recurrent theme in this approach to the understanding of eating disorders. Some have regarded anorexia as an act of extreme compliance or conformity, others as an act of defiance and rebellion. The latter view is probably the more common, it is powerfully presented by psychotherapist Susie Orbach in her 1986 book *Hunger Strike*. Orbach writes: 'In trying to come to grips with anorexia I have encounted a formidable strength and determination in individual women which allowed one to understand how much of the anorexia is both an honourable protest and profoundly worthy cause.' I will examine these views in more detail in chapter 3, here we may note we have come full circle, as we have returned to the theme of protest.

Just as the behaviour of Indian ascetics or the suffragettes can be understood not in terms of illness (though they may certainly become ill through lack of food), but in terms of their social and cultural context, their aspirations and goals, or beliefs and desires, so too anorexia and bulimia it is claimed, can be understood if we examine the social context in which it occurs, and the individual experience of the women involved.

Summary

What are anorexia and bulimia? In this chapter we have looked at various forms of self-imposed starvation. Such behaviour demands an explanation in view of the common response to food shortages, and the fear of starvation, which has been only too common throughout human history. We noted examples of self-starvation, or fasting, which may be understood as a form of human action, a product of individual choice, with specific motivation and identifiable objectives. In this respect there is no essential difference between these behaviours and other more familiar human actions such as, for example, getting married.

From the seventeenth century medical authorities began to identify a condition of severe emaciation that could not be attributed to any known physical disease. It seemed that the emaciation had been brought about through voluntary restriction of food intake; the starvation had been self-induced. However, there seemed to be no justification for the self-starvation in terms of, for example, religious or political aspirations.

In the absence of physical disease, and in the absence of plausible justification, the condition inevitably came to be classified as a form of mental illness. Our usual understanding of illness is that it is not a form of action, it is a natural event. Illness is more like growing old than getting married. Illnesses are not things we do, but things we get. To claim that these examples of self-starvation are fundamentally, that is qualitatively, different from say a political hunger strike and should be regarded as illnesses, raises considerable problems. As we have seen this 'peculiar form of disease' has provided medical authorities, keen to understand and classify the condition, with serious difficulties over the last 100 years or so. Anorexia nervosa has been identified with every major category of psychiatric disorder, as well as being regarded as a physical illness, and has even been dismissed as non-existent.

But despite the problems most people would accept that anorexia nervosa is an illness. When a severely emaciated anorexic tells you she is 'too fat', and feels 'disgusted' with herself for having eaten half a spoonful more food than she 'should', it is difficult to believe that we are dealing with essentially the same phenomenon as, say, a politically motivated hunger strike. And yet there is certainly considerable discomfort in regarding anorexia nervosa as an illness. The anorexic, at least in the earlier stages of the condition, appears to be engaged in a deliberate, purposeful, and even rational activity. Early on her beliefs and desires concerning body weight are indistinguishable from those of most women in Western cultures.

Some writers have cautiously accepted that anorexia may be an illness, but have argued that it is an illness with a very special cultural significance. It is a form of mental disturbance intimately related to a specific social context, in particular it may express the contradictions and discomforts of being a woman in Western culture. Advocates of this position may reject the illness classification altogether, and argue anorexia is fundamentally the same as a political hunger strike, and stands as a symbol of, and a protest against, the oppression of women in our society.

It would appear that anorexia nervosa does not fit comfortably into any classification. It is hoped that this chapter has shown that anorexia nervosa is a puzzling condition which raises very considerable problems for anyone attempting to think seriously about it. Many of the issues touched on in this chapter will be considered in more detail in chapters 2, 3 and 4.

2 Identifying anorexia and bulimia

Anorexia nervosa

Case example

Elizabeth has a successful career in ballet. She is 25 years old and deeply committed to her work. She has lived away from her parents for the last seven years, but has frequent contact with them. Her father is a solicitor and her mother a university lecturer. Elizabeth has no brothers or sisters. Six months ago she went to her GP to ask for sleeping tablets. She had been having difficulty sleeping for the previous four months and was finding her work schedule exhausting. At this time Elizabeth weighed five and a half stone. Her GP was concerned, as she appeared to have lost a lot of weight since he last saw her three months previously. Elizabeth pointed out she had always been thin, and that her weight was normal for someone in her career. After obtaining more information on her sleep pattern, attitude and mood, her GP concluded Elizabeth was suffering from depression and prescribed anti-depressants. He was not entirely reassured about her weight so arranged to see her in a month. A month later she was unchanged. Due to work commitments she could not see him again for two months. On this third visit she looked exhausted and considerably thinner than on any previous visit. She had lost a further seven pounds, making her weight 60% of the average expected weight for a woman of her age and height. Admission to hospital was considered but Elizabeth's insistence that she would co-operate with an out-patient programme led to her referral for out-patient treatment.

'I just can't keep up at work, I feel tired all the time ... people are talking as if the problem is that I don't eat enough. But that isn't it, something is going wrong at work, it's just not like it used to be, but I'm trying to put it right. I was too heavy, that was making the work difficult, I could see the others were getting better parts because they were thinner and more energetic than me. I've tried my best to get some of my weight off, but

I'm not there yet ... It's difficult, sometimes I feel so hungry, but I have to be really careful. If I could just get my weight to the right level I'm sure everything would be fine. If only I weren't so fat, you should see the others, they are much thinner than me. Its terrible.'

Case example

Sarah was referred by her GP, she is 19 and has recently returned home from university. She has completed two terms of her first year, and has decided not to continue with her degree. She had been referred a year previously but did not attend. At that time she was preparing for her 'A' levels. Her family, particularly her mother, had become concerned about her refusal to eat with them. At first this was explained by Sarah as her needing the time to study. She would take her meals to her room. However, her mother noticed very little of the food was eaten, she realised Sarah was flushing much of it down the toilet. Her weight began to fall. Sarah insisted that she was alright and that once the exams were over she would be fine. Despite her anxieties her mother went along with this, and did not press her to attend her appointment. After her 'A' levels Sarah spent the summer away from home working at a children's camp. She returned just before she was due to start her first year at university. After her first term she returned for the Christmas break. She had lost more weight. Fierce arguments about food kept occurring, especially over Christmas itself. On two occasions Sarah's mother heard her being sick in the toilet. To placate her mother Sarah said she would see the doctor at the university, 'just to check', although she insisted she felt fine. By the Easter break Sarah's weight had fallen still further, and on her return home she told her parents of her decision not to continue with her degree. Sarah now weighs six stone three pounds, which is 65% of her average expected body weight. She has not menstruated for nine months.

Sarah's father is a successful business man, who because of a prolonged illness had spent a lot of time with Sarah in her early years. He had great hopes of her, especially as her two elder sisters had 'let him down' by not going to university. He is now furious at Sarah's 'wilfulness', and has 'washed his hands' of her. As Sarah talks about her father she sits on the edge of her chair, getting as close to the radiator as she can. Her fingers have a blueish tinge. She keeps her heavy coat, scarf and hat on.

'People don't seem to realise I feel alright. Everything would be fine if they just left me alone.' At university she had gone swimming every day, and had played tennis twice a week: 'So how can I be ill?' Sarah had gradually withdrawn from social contacts because even her friends had kept on about her weight. At times she felt they were jealous because she could resist food when they couldn't. But sometimes she would give in and eat everything she could find. After these binges she would panic and make sure she ate even less in the following week. Then she discovered she could get rid of the food quickly and easily by vomiting. 'It seems to solve everything, if I do lose control and eat I can at least prevent putting on any weight.' Even so she describes such loss of control as 'letting herself down' and feels 'disgusted' with herself for being so 'weak and worthless'. To compensate she would eat less and do more exercise the next day. She described this as 'fighting back' and 'winning' after the earlier 'setback'. When she is 'winning' in this way she feels in control and has proved to the world that she is special, different, and superior to everyone else. She describes a vast gulf between herself and others. No one understood, and she didn't want to have to explain. 'If only people would stop hounding me ... '

Diagnosis. What aspects of these descriptions would lead to a diagnosis of anorexia nervosa? Over the last 20 years various sets of diagnostic criteria have been proposed, and although there is no universally accepted definition there is a reasonable consensus on the type of features significant for diagnosis. The six points listed below provide an outline of the core, or essential, characteristics of anorexia nervosa:

1 Weight loss of at least 25% of original body weight (or weight 25% below the average expected for one's sex, age, and height).
2 Amenorrhoea (i.e. loss of menstruation).
3 No known physical illness that would account for the weight loss.
4 Refusal to maintain a minimal expected body weight for one's sex, age, and height.
5 Intense fear of gaining weight, or becoming fat, which does not diminish with weight loss.
6 Disturbance in the way in which one's body weight, size, or shape is experienced (e.g. claiming to 'feel fat', even when emaciated).

These six features will be the prime focus of a doctor's investigation when considering a diagnosis of anorexia nervosa. It may be noted that although anorexia nervosa means 'loss of appetite of nervous origin', in fact loss of appetite is not an identifying feature of the condition. On the contrary many anorexics report experiencing intense hunger which they have to battle against in order to maintain their low weight. Diagnostically significant physical signs are primarily severe weight loss and amenorrhoea. But there will usually be other physical signs and symptoms of starvation, the following are the most frequently reported:

bradycardia (slow heart beat)
hypotension (low blood pressure)
hypothermia (lowered body temperature)
sensitivity to cold
acrocyanosis (blueish-mauve extremities: hands, feet, nose, and
   ears)
pallid face
lanugo hair (growth of soft downy hair on parts of the body that are
   normally hairless, especially hands, face and back)
constipation
oedema (retention of body fluid)
muscle wasting
physical weakness
dizziness
restlessness
insomnia
hyperactivity
reduction in sexual responsiveness
resistance to infection.

These physical signs and symptoms are the result of starvation. They are therefore not unique to anorexia nervosa: anyone subjected to a prolonged and severe reduction in food intake (for whatever reason) will undergo similar physical changes. It is therefore essential that a physician considers other possible causes of weight loss before making a diagnosis of anorexia nervosa (as noted in point 3 of the six essential features of the condition given above).

The most obvious physical sign of anorexia nervosa is, of course, severe weight loss. Amenorrhoea, or cessation of menstruation, is another important feature of the condition. As a general guide, if weight continues to fall to a level approximately 85% of expected average weight (which is calculated on the basis of sex, age, and height), menstruation is likely to stop. Although there is a disagreement as to why amenorrhoea occurs in anorexia nervosa the evidence favours the view that it occurs as a result of changes in hormone levels brought on by starvation. Many of the other signs and symptoms listed above are related to a general slowing down of the chemical processes occurring in the body, that is through a reduction in metabolic rate. When food intake is severely restricted, and weight falls, the body will start to use up reserves of nutrients which have been stored in the body. The reduction in metabolic rate allows the body to conserve increasingly scarce resources. As a result less heat is generated, and blood is diverted away from the skin and extremities to central organs like the brain. These changes lead to a number of the signs and symptoms listed above, for example: slow heart beat, low blood pressure, lowered body temperature, blueish-mauve extremities, and sensitivity to cold.

The growth of thin downy hair (termed lanugo hair) on parts of the body which are normally hairless (notably the face, shoulders and back), may be part of the body's attempt to conserve heat. Constipation occurs when the body attempts to draw required levels of fluid from very small amounts of food. This process produces hard dry pellets which are difficult for the intestine to move and are difficult to pass. This problem can be eased by drinking more fluids, but as this will show as weight increase on scales, and can lead to an uncomfortable feeling of fullness, many anorexics put strict limits on fluid intake as well as food intake. Muscle wasting occurs when, due to dramatic reductions of body fat, the body begins to break down the protein in muscles to use as fuel. Eventually this leads to a reduction in physical strength, and an inability to sustain physical activity.

It has often been noted that anorexics are highly resistant to infectious diseases. Why this should be so is not clear. It appears that in some way the reduction in metabolic rate creates an environment within the body unfavourable for the activity of the organisms responsible for infectious diseases. However, while the anorexic appears to be less vulnerable to illnesses such as the common cold, there should be no doubt that anorexia nervosa is a serious condition that can be fatal. For example heart or kidney failure can occur as a result of potassium depletion. Also in addition to restricting food intake anorexics may try to lose weight through other means, for example, abuse of laxatives (an anorexic may consume up to 100 laxatives per day), use of diuretics (to increase the passing of water), vomiting, and vigorous exercise. Such activities can lead to further physical complications, which will be outlined in the section below on bulimia. Once weight begins to increase and a more adequate diet is established these physical changes will generally be reversed.

The physical signs associated with anorexia are the result of self-imposed starvation. This deliberate food restriction is prompted by a distinctive attitude to body shape and weight, and it is this characteristic attitude that is referred to in points four to six of our list of core features given above. This psychological characteristic is absolutely essential to the diagnosis and without this distinctive attitude to weight gain the diagnosis would not be made (without the presence of this attitude a physician is likely to diagnosis the condition as 'secondary', or 'pseudo' anorexia nervosa). This characteristic feature involves extreme concerns about shape and weight, and is often referred to as the 'anorexic attitude'. There have been a number of highly influential accounts attempting to describe the features of the 'anorexic attitude'. Professor A. Crisp of St George's Hospital, London, has described it as a 'morbid fear of pubescent weight'. Crisp suggests that it is specifically the weight associated with sexual maturity that is feared by the anorexic, low weight serving to stave off menstruation and changes in body shape which occur with sexual development. Crisp has also offered the more general description: 'weight phobia'. Gerald Russell suggests a similar description: 'a morbid fear of fatness'. American psychiatrist Hilde Bruch considers the 'anorexic attitude' to centre on a 'relentless pursuit of thinness'. The term 'relentless' vividly captures the overriding preoccupation that body weight comes to have in the life of the anorexic.

The anorexic comes to subordinate every other concern to a central preoccupation with controlling food intake in order to lose weight. If conflicts arise between this 'relentless' pursuit of thinness, and other concerns such as career, friendships or family, the pursuit of thinness will come first. The prospect of overeating and gaining weight becomes a source of intense anxiety and extreme discomfort. As this preoccupation progresses the anorexic's sense of self-worth, or self-esteem, will come to be intimately bound up with her weight and food intake. Any increase in body weight is both feared and seen as repugnant. Anorexics will often describe body fat as 'revolting' or 'disgusting'. Body weight often comes to be seen in moral terms: fatness being morally reprehensible, while thinness is regarded, not only as desirable, but also as morally praiseworthy. Thinness confers moral superiority. A persistent and pervasive self-judgement occurs solely on the basis of weight control. Weight increases or loss of control of eating may provoke severe self-criticism and depression, anorexics will often say they are 'disgusted' with themselves for having lost control. Where control of food intake and loss of weight is occurring there is often a feeling of triumph and euphoria. These emotional changes will often hinge exclusively on current food intake and weight, while other life events seem comparatively unimportant. This central feature of anorexia nervosa clearly involves a crisis of identity. The difficulties with which the anorexic appears to be struggling are often referred to as 'existential' problems. That is, the anorexic appears to be engaged in a struggle to establish a sense of individual identity, of self-worth, and of autonomy and control over her life. This she attempts to do through control of body shape and weight, an activity that is experienced by the anorexic as a solution to these 'existential' problems. Being thin, being in control, offers sense of identity and value apparently unobtainable through other means.

A prominent feature of the psychological aspects of anorexia nervosa is distortion of body image (point 6 in the above list of central features of anorexia). The most striking distortion is in terms of how the anorexic experiences her body. Often she will describe herself as overweight, and say she 'feels fat', even when dangerously emaciated. But in addition to experiencing themselves as fat, anorexics will often say they look fat when they see themselves in a mirror. A number of studies have looked at this latter feature. One method of studying this is to project through a special lens a photograph of the person onto a screen. The lens can distort the image by 20%, making the subject appear fatter or thinner. Subjects are asked to adjust the image so that it accurately reflects how they are, and also how they would like to be.

With this technique results indicate about 35% of anorexics overestimate their body size by more than 10%, while only 5% of normal weight women do. Further this distortion appears to be found only in relation to themselves, not when they estimated size of other people or objects. However, this work has been questioned and it has been argued that there is little difference in the extent of body misperception between anorexics and non-anorexics.

Weight loss can occur as a result of other psychological disturbances such as depression. In practice, weight loss associated with anorexia nervosa may be identified when the central features of intense fear of fatness and distortions of body image are present. In the case of Sarah and Elizabeth the presence of these core features would lead to a diagnosis of anorexia nervosa. Sarah is probably close to the stereotype, particularly with regard to her family conflicts. But as we have seen these are not defining characteristics. In Elizabeth's case the diagnosis relied almost entirely on identifying the 'anorexic attitude', because her low weight, lack of menstruation and dietary restrictions, are not particularly unusual in the distinctive subculture of ballet.

Between 90 and 95% of those receiving the diagnosis of anorexia nervosa are female. Most anorexics are between 16 and 35 years of age, although 'atypical anorexia nervosa' can occur at any age. Some sources make a distinction between post-pubertal anorexia nervosa (arising after puberty) and pre-menarchal anorexia nervosa (where the condition begins before the girl has started to menstruate).

Bulimia nervosa

Case example
Clare is a 21-year-old music student in the final year of her degree. She and her partner Jonathan have lived in a small flat for the last two years. He is also studying music. Clare entered therapy at the insistence of Jonathan. She had been treated for depression when she was 19, and had been in therapy for six months when she was 14 after she had been diagnosed as

suffering from anorexia nervosa. Clare has an elder brother and sister. Her sister now lives in Australia. Clare is very worried about her brother, who has been addicted to heroin for many years, and despite various forms of therapy has not managed to become free of the drug for longer than a few months at a time.

Clare describes her relationship to her mother and father as close, but she feels that in the past they have asked too much of her and of her brother. 'We could never satisfy them. We were never quite good enough.' Both parents have had successful careers in teaching. Clare had been bingeing for the previous year. Her weight was just below that expected for her age and height. 'I've always had a big appetite, even when I lost a lot of weight when I was 14. It was a major discovery: realising I could eat what I wanted without getting fat. Eating makes me feel better, it seems to block things out: hunger, anger, loneliness, everything. But of course afterwards I was horrified at the thought of getting fatter. A friend of mine told me she binged and kept slim by vomiting afterwards, that's when it started. Being sick keeps me in charge, without that I would be completely out of control.' Clare describes a cycle of bingeing, generally on large quantities of select foods (e.g. four pounds of cheese, four large tubs of yoghurt, six apples, etc.) followed by vomiting. This will be followed by several days of complete abstinence from food, during which she feels depressed and guilty. Once she starts to eat again she becomes preoccupied with the next binge. This cycle has come to dominate her life. She desperately wanted to keep her behaviour secret, especially from her partner. She felt deeply ashamed when he discovered what she was doing, and agreed to enter therapy largely to please him.

Case example
Kathy is a 25-year-old nurse. She lives at home with her mother and younger brother. Her mother and father divorced when she was 12. She is engaged to Mark, who is 30 and works as an electrician. They are saving to buy a house, and hope to start a family as soon as they are married. Kathy has a wide circle of friends and enjoys meeting people and going out, especially to parties. She takes great care of her appearance and is of expected weight for her age and height. 'Ever since I was little I have been heavier than I would like to be. As I grew older I tried

to diet but I hated it. I enjoy eating you see. How can you enjoy a night out if you have to watch everything you eat?' Kathy describes her feelings before a binge. 'I know when I'm going to do it, hours – sometimes days – before. It's a kind of relief when I've stopped avoiding it, somehow I stop worrying about things. I plan it carefully. I make sure everyone will be out and I stock up on food. I have spent up to £100 on food for a binge. I buy all the things I normally avoid, cakes, biscuits, sweets ... anything. I've read some people just eat food they know they can bring up easily. But for me eating and being sick is a release, I don't have to care anymore. So, all the brakes are off. I eat anything, whatever catches my eye I'll buy it. You see I know I can get rid of it. After the binge, I'm sick and it's like being set free. I'm exhausted but I feel I've got rid of it all, and I'm alright, relaxed. After a while I feel disgusted with myself ... It's just like waking up with a hangover.' Kathy sought professional help after reading about the physical dangers that can result from bulimia, and finding herself completely unable to prevent the cycle of bingeing and vomiting that had continued for two years.

Diagnosis. What are the features of these accounts that would indicate a diagnosis of bulimia nervosa? The core features of the condition are as follows:

1 Recurrent episodes of 'binge eating' (i.e. rapid consumption of a large amount of food in a discrete period of time).
2 A feeling of lack of control over eating behaviour during the eating binges.
3 The person regularly engages in purges (i.e. self-induced vomiting, use of laxatives or diuretics, strict dieting or fasting, or vigorous exercise) in order to prevent weight gain.
4 A minimum average of two binge eating episodes a week for at least three months.
5 Persistent over-concern with body shape and weight.

The central feature of bulimia is binge eating, that is, the consumption of large amounts of food in relatively brief periods of time. The average daily intake for an adult in a Western society is 1,500 to 2,000 calories per day; in a single binge a bulimic may consume 50,000 calories. What is regarded as a binge varies enormously; some people consider eating an extra biscuit to be a binge, while others would consider themselves to have binged after having eaten the equivalent of two or three main meals. However, a crucial feature of bulimia nervosa is a feeling of one's eating behaviour being out of control (the second point in the above list). The frequency of binge eating can vary from once a month to 20 times a day or more. Point 4 in the above list indicates the level of severity that will usually be present before a diagnosis will be made. Bulimia is sometimes referred to as the 'binge-purge syndrome', and, as point 3 of our list notes, purging can take various forms. Typically purging is done through vomiting after eating, but other forms of purging include use of laxatives, diuretics, enemas, diet pills, drug use, severe food restriction, and vigorous exercise. Purging frequently has the function not just of ridding the body of food (and hence avoiding weight gain), but also of removing unwanted feelings such as anxiety, panic, guilt, and tension.

Bulimia has at times been compared to an addiction. Some have suggested the addiction is to food, but others that the addiction is to vomiting or purging. In either case the behaviour becomes compulsive and the individual reports being unable to prevent it. In both Clare's and Kathy's descriptions there is an emphasis on the purging aspect as a release from tension. However another essential feature for the diagnosis is, as in the case of anorexia, the fifth point listed above: a distinctive attitude to body weight and shape. Anorexics and bulimics share similar psychological characteristics. Bulimics have a similar fear of fatness, preoccupation with body shape and weight, polarised attitudes towards thinness and fatness, and distortion of body image. Despite the striking physical difference – the bulimic will usually be at or near normal weight and be menstruating normally – the two conditions are linked by distinctive attitudes to weight and body shape. Both will come to regard their self-worth as being intricately bound up with their food intake and body shape. This crucial similarity has led many authorities to regard bulimia as a variation of anorexia.

Although there has been less disagreement about the definition or diagnosis of bulimia, there has been a great deal of debate on the issue of the relationship between anorexia and bulimia. It has been argued that bulimia is the end stage of anorexia, but this is doubtful in view of studies which suggest below 50% of bulimics have had a previous history of anorexia. The experience of Clare, who was treated for anorexia eight years before presenting with bulimia is therefore not typical. In the case of Sarah we noted she was also caught in a cycle of bingeing and purging. Hence she would fulfil the diagnostic criteria for both anorexia and bulimia. In such cases anorexia is the diagnosis made, as bulimia is currently regarded as a variant or sub-group of anorexia. Evidence indicates that between 40 and 50% of anorexics have episodes of bulimia.

Differentiation

We can therefore differentiate four types:

1 Anorexia nervosa – restrictive or 'classical'.
2 Anorexia nervosa – with bulimic episodes.
3 Normal weight bulimia with history of anorexia nervosa.
4 Normal weight bulimia without history of anorexia nervosa.

Elizabeth would be an example of restrictive anorexia, and Sarah of anorexia with bulimic episodes. Clare presents with normal weight bulimia with a history of anorexia, and Kathy normal weight bulimia without a history of anorexia. In terms of response to therapy, types 1 and 4 are usually more responsive than types 2 and 3.

These distinctions are made on the basis of the crucial features of body weight, and the presence or absence of bingeing and purging. All four will be linked by the distinctive 'anorexic attitude'. As we can see this term is not particularly appropriate as this distinctive attitude characterises bulimia as well as anorexia. Some have argued bulimics may be regarded as 'failed' anorexics. However, it should be noted that considerable disagreement still surrounds the relationship between anorexia and bulimia.

We have been discussing what is usually termed 'case-level' anorexia and bulimia. That is, we have considered the sorts of features which must be present before a diagnosis of anorexia or bulimia will be made. But surveys suggest anorexic or bulimic behaviour is very common in the general population, though not severe enough to warrant the diagnosis. We will consider this in the next section.

'The tip of an iceberg'?

Studies of the prevalence of anorexia among secondary school girls in England indicates between 0.5 and 1% fulfil the diagnostic criteria. The prevalence of bulimia among female British students has been found to be about 13%, and among the general population about 2%. However, it is often remarked in the literature that the number of people actually fulfilling these strict diagnostic criteria is merely the 'tip of an iceberg'. It is claimed that there are large numbers of people with problems similar to anorexia or bulimia who do not fulfil the strict 'case-level' criteria. Is this true?

A number of studies have identified women who experience similar preoccupations with body weight and shape, and engage in behaviours characteristic of anorexia but do so without extreme weight loss. The term 'subclinical anorexia nervosa' has been suggested for this group. The prevalence of subclinical anorexia in student populations appears to be about 5%. In similar populations, studies have found a prevalence of what might be termed 'subclinical bulimia' as high as 20%. It appears that most cases of subclinical anorexia and bulimia do not become severe enough to meet the diagnostic criteria. Ingvar Nyladen, a Swedish psychiatrist, suggests: 'Most cases of anorexia nervosa are incipient and/or mild and never come to medical attention but are spontaneously cured'.

It has been argued that anorexia occurs on a continuum with the minority who develop the full-blown condition at one end, and what might be regarded as a normal concern with dieting and weight control at the other. The differences between the various points on the continuum, from normal dieting to subclinical or incipient forms, through to mild and severe 'case-level' anorexia, would then be simply a difference of degree. If this is true anorexia may be regarded as essentially normal preoccupations with weight that have got out of control. David Garner (a psychologist working in Canada) and his colleagues present a more complex picture in their discussion of the continuum view. Put briefly, their research suggests that some features identified in the diagnostic criteria do occur on a continuum, whereas other features are specific to the disorder. They argue the preoccupation with weight, weight loss, dietary behaviour, etc., appears to occur on a continuum which includes 'normal dieters' and 'case level' anorexia. However, anorexia nervosa can be distinguished from dietary preoccupation (or 'normal' concerns with weight) by quite specific psychological traits. For example, they identify a sense of personal ineffectiveness, unawareness of internal states, and interpersonal distrust. The crucial point is that the underlying motivation for engaging in weight control appears to differ in anorexic and non-anorexic groups. This suggests that it would be easy to over-diagnose on the basis of dietary behaviour and emphasises the point made above of the central feature of diagnosis being the identification of a characteristic attitude.

Similar discussions have occurred with respect to bulimia in view of the very large numbers of people who engage in overeating and purging. Recently publications focusing on 'social bulimia', or 'fad bulimia', have suggested that on some American college campuses as many as 50% of women have engaged in group bingeing and vomiting sessions. The argument has been advanced that, just as weight control through dieting and exercising is normal in our society, so too vomiting after a heavy meal is in fact normal practice for many people. Frequent vomiting, especially if habitually followed by periods of severe restriction of food intake, can be very dangerous. Complications include: increased blood pressure, severe electrolyte imbalance in body cells, urinary infections, renal failure, epileptic seizures, potassium depletion, dental decay, haemorrhaging, heart strain, etc. But it is claimed the occasional use of vomiting as a means of weight control entails less risk than, say, smoking, and is in fact very widely practised.

Studies which have attempted to assess the extent of eating problems have generally focused on specific populations, such as college or university students, or within particular careers such as dancing and modelling. However some studies of the general population have been carried out, one of which was published by psychologist Peter Cooper and his colleagues in 1984. Their survey of a sample of the general population in England involved 369 women aged between 15 and 40, with the majority (63%) being in their twenties: 20.6% of these women reported they had an eating problem. The two factors most strongly associated with reporting an eating problem were: episodes of binge eating and a high score on a questionnaire (The Eating Attitudes Test), which measures the extent of concern about weight and food intake. As many as 80-90% habitually exercise control over their eating. There seems to be little doubt that concerns about body shape and weight, and anxieties about eating are very widespread among women in our society.

Summary

In this chapter we have reviewed the core characteristics, or central identifying features, of anorexia and bulimia. These are the essential features that will be looked for when a diagnosis of anorexia or bulimia is being considered. As we have seen, in addition to the core features listed in the diagnostic criteria there are many other characteristics indicative of the condition which also help identification. However, it must be emphasised that a clear-cut identification is not always easy. As we have seen, certain features of anorexia and bulimia are extremely common in our society. Concerns about weight and dieting, or instances of bingeing and vomiting, are not in themselves sufficient to warrant a diagnosis of anorexia or bulimia. It is common for parents to assume a family member has an eating disorder when in fact they are displaying 'normal' concerns with shape and weight. On the other hand, parents may at times deny what they are seeing and refuse to believe what is happening to their daughter. The problem of early identification, and the important question: 'At what point should professional opinion be sought?', will be addressed in chapter 5.

In conclusion I would like to emphasise the point made in the preface to this book. In presenting information on factors likely to lead to a diagnosis of anorexia or bulimia, the object of the exercise is to assess whether difficulties associated with eating and weight have reached a point where professional help is required. Applying labels is not an end in itself, and can often be extremely unhelpful if the label provokes stereotyped thinking and responses.

3 What causes anorexia and bulimia?

Anorexia nervosa is a condition of self-imposed starvation. The emaciation characteristic of the condition is not the result of a physical abnormality or disease. The anorexic deliberately starves herself. As we have seen in chapter 2 the central feature of the diagnosis is the identification of a particular attitude to body weight. This attitude involves intense fear of weight gain and specific distortions in body image (e.g. feeling fat when emaciated). The anorexic is emaciated because she has decided, quite consciously and deliberately, to restrict her food intake in order to reduce her body weight. Bulimia nervosa, though not characterised by severe weight loss, also often involves periods of self-starvation which alternate with bouts of binge eating and purging. How are we to explain this behaviour? When we classify a piece of behaviour as a conscious or deliberate action, explanations which give information about beliefs or desires are usually sufficient. Hence a question such as why did Gautama Siddhartha starve himself to the point of extreme emaciation will usually be explained in terms of his religious beliefs and aspirations (as outlined in chapter 1). An important variation of this type of explanation may be presented by those influenced by psychoanalytic writings in which behaviour may be explained in terms of unconscious impulses and motivations.

A person with anorexia or bulimia has certain beliefs, and desires, centring around her body shape and weight. And in a sense these beliefs and desires do explain her behaviour. If you believe being fat is revolting, perhaps even wicked, you will want to be thin and do all you can to avoid becoming fat. It appears that the anorexic's behaviour does follow logically from the 'anorexic attitude', i.e. her beliefs and desires. What is the difference between the beliefs and desires motivating the anorexic or bulimic and, say, those motivating a religious ascetic? Why do we accept that the beliefs and desires of the ascetic are legitimate explanations of their behaviour, but reject the explanations offered by anorexics? Two crucial differences have been suggested: first, the beliefs and desires of the anorexic appear grossly distorted or exaggerated; and, second, anorexics and bulimics appear not to be able to change their behaviour, that is, their behaviour has features of a compulsion or addiction. Obviously we want to know more than her conscious beliefs or desires when we ask: 'Why does she starve herself?' Hence it is not just the act of starvation that we want to explain, it is also the attitude which underlies it. That is, the reasons the anorexic gives for her behaviour are part of the problem to be explained. How does she come to see the world and herself as she does? How does a pattern of thought and behaviour which can be lethal, develop?

In discussions of the aetiology (or 'assigning of cause') of anorexia nervosa we encounter considerable controversy. We noted in chapter 1 that it has been extremely difficult to classify this behaviour. What is it? A physical illness, or a mental illness? A protest? A political statement? Clearly the way we view (or classify) the condition will determine the sort of causes we look for. To put it crudely, if anorexia is essentially a protest the crucial causal factors will be the conditions which the behaviour is protesting against and the beliefs and desires of the individual making the protest.

Just as there have been various ways of classifying anorexia and bulimia there have been various attempts at identifying the cause. The fact is that we do not know the precise cause, or causes, of anorexia nervosa or bulimia nervosa. However there is a wide range of evidence pointing to a number of factors which appear to be of aetiological significance. Current evidence suggests that anorexia and bulimia are caused by the complex interaction and timing of a wide range of contributory factors. In this and the following chapter I will present a model of anorexia and bulimia which views them as conditions with multiple determinants. This model is based on the work of David Garner (a psychologist) and Paul Garfinkel (a psychiatrist), both working in Canada. When considering the multiple determinants of anorexia and bulimia we may organise our thinking by dividing causes into: (a) predisposing factors (i.e. conditions which increase an individual's vulnerability to develop the disorder), (b) precipitating factors (i.e. conditions which may trigger the condition), and (c) perpetuating factors (i.e. conditions which seem to maintain or prolong the disorder).

In this chapter we will consider the various determinants of anorexia and bulimia under these three headings, as in the following outline:

Predisposing factors:
    Individual characteristics
    Family characteristics (this will be covered in chapter 4)
    Socio-cultural factors.

Precipitating factors:
    Various forms of stress including:
    Achievement pressure
    Difficulties or conflicts surrounding sex
    Separation, loss or bereavement
    Socio-economic change
    Dieting and weight loss.

Perpetuating factors:
    The psychological effects of starvation
    Various forms of reinforcement.

Predisposing factors

Individual characteristics. What kinds of people develop anorexia or bulimia? Is it possible to identify a particular type of personality who is likely, or at least at risk of, developing anorexia? Many descriptions of the personalities of anorexics and bulimics have been published.

Anorexics are frequently described as being: obsessional, hysterical, egocentric, introspective, introverted, shy, emotionally immature, irritable, hostile, moody, unsociable, socially anxious, obstinate, manipulative, deceitful, wilful, compliant, over-dependent on family, approval seeking, perfectionist, inhibited, highly intelligent, competitive, superior, self-critical, aloof, etc.

Descriptions of bulimics often involve qualities such as: indulgent, impulsive, compulsive, seductive, disorganised, chaotic, outgoing, sociable, emotionally unstable, dishonest, tendency to abuse drugs, dependent, compliant, conforming, uncontrolled, weak, depressive, unassertive, over-sensitive, approval seeking, etc.

Two questions arise from these descriptions:

1 Do these descriptions really identify a characteristic anorexic or bulimic personality?

2 Do these descriptions provide us with an outline of the type of personality predisposed to develop anorexia or bulimia?

Concerning the first question, research has demonstrated that there is considerable variation in personality among both anorexics and bulimics. However, some personality characteristics do appear to be significantly associated with these conditions. For example, obsessive-compulsive tendencies, introversion, and general anxiety, are common among anorexics. Tendency to depression and to act impulsively appears to be common among bulimics.

However, concerning the second question, it is very important to note that profound changes in personality occur in the course of the development of anorexia and bulimia, hence we cannot infer from descriptions of people with these conditions a predisposing personality type. It is in fact very difficult to obtain an accurate picture of 'pre-morbid' personality. However, evidence, such as it is, does suggest that some personality traits of anorexics and bulimics may be significant in the development of the illness, and hence predate onset, and persist after recovery. These include an intense need for approval from others, a tendency to conformity, conscientiousness, perfectionism, obsessionality, and a lack of responsiveness to inner needs. A typical childhood profile of someone likely to develop anorexia is one of a well-behaved, introverted, and conscientious child. There is often evidence of a considerable amount of self-discipline and ability to apply themselves, for example to academic work. It is of course this capacity for conscientious determined effort, when focused on control of body weight, that characterises anorexia nervosa.

In popular accounts of anorexia nervosa one often reads that the anorexic is someone who refuses to grow up, and that self-starvation is a means of avoiding sexual maturity. The British psychiatrist Arthur Crisp has written extensively about the role of sexuality in the development of anorexia nervosa. The start of menstruation and the emergence of secondary sexual characteristics are dependent on the presence of a specific level of body fat. Hence for adolescent females the emergence of sexuality and increased body fat are crucially related. Crisp notes the reduction of body weight to a pre-pubertal level allows the individual to avoid the maturational demands associated with puberty. Hence, while the signs and symptoms of anorexia nervosa focus on eating and body weight, the condition essentially expresses a profound underlying resistance (which may be more or less unconscious) to sexual and psychological maturity. It should be noted that while some advocates of this view consider weight loss to be prompted by an unconscious fear of psycho-sexual maturity, Crisp has suggested that initially the motive to lose weight may be identical to the non-anorexic. However, the anorexic finds the 'turning off' of puberty a relief and as a result develops an intense aversion, or 'phobia', towards increased body weight. Strictly speaking then, on this latter view, the avoidance of the adjustment demands of puberty is a reward, hence a factor that maintains the condition. It appears to be the case that certain people are predisposed to find puberty particularly threatening. Crisp notes that anorexics are significantly heavier at birth, develop secondary sexual characteristics and begin menstruating earlier than non-anorexics. It would follow from this that the individual experiences a premature demand for sexual adjustment. Another factor which may heighten the adjustment demands at puberty is a family background of discomfort and anxiety surrounding sexuality.

The American psychiatrist Hilde Bruch has made a major contribution to the understanding of anorexia nervosa. She has focused on the development of psychological functioning in the context of the family, with particular emphasis on the early mother-daughter relationship (this will be discussed in more detail in chapter 4). She has argued that the defining characteristic of anorexia, the 'relentless pursuit of thinness', is the outcome of: 'a desperate fight against feeling enslaved and exploited', the anorexic is struggling against the idea that she is 'not competent to lead a life of her own'. She considers anorexia nervosa to be a 'development impasse', in which 'the main issue is a struggle for control, for a sense of identity, competence and effectiveness'. The condition develops, according to Bruch, in the context of years of struggle to be perfect, it is an expression of the individual's 'paralysing sense of ineffectiveness', in the face of perfectionist performance demands. Bruch has emphasised three areas of disturbed psychological functioning which she believes pre-date the development of the illness:

1 Perceptual disturbances involving severe distortions of body image.
2 Conceptual disturbances which lead to misinterpretations of internal and external cues, especially with regard to the identification of needs (e.g. of hunger).
3 An underlying, paralysing sense of ineffectiveness.

Although there is some evidence that anorexics and bulimics do experience these disturbances it is not clear that such problems are unique to anorexia and bulimia or that they clearly pre-date onset of the illness. Bruch's account of the origin of these three disturbances focuses on the early relationship between mother and child. Bruch has also suggested that apart from the three specific areas noted above anorexics and bulimics have wide-ranging 'disturbances in conceptualisation'. She has argued that they retain the thinking styles of young children. She believes these deficits are a consequence of early experiences which lead to a failure of maturation. Hence, she claims this feature pre-dates and is a predisposing factor in the development of the illness.

Investigations into the disturbances in thinking present in anorexia and bulimia have drawn on the work of the American psychiatrist A. T. Beck who has identified six types of 'faulty information processing', or 'cognitive distortions', which are present in various forms of emotional disturbance. In the following list I have given some examples of how these distortions manifest in anorexia and bulimia.

1 **Arbitrary inference:** involves forming a conclusion when there is little or no supporting evidence, or even when the evidence clearly contradicts the conclusion.
Examples:
   'If I eat an extra biscuit it will make me fat.'
   'If I can lose more weight everything will be fine.'
   'If someone says I look well, they mean I look fat.'

2 **Selective abstraction:** involves focusing exclusively on one aspect of a situation and ignoring other features.
Examples:
   'When I'm thin I'm special.'
   'The only time I am happy is when I'm thin.'
   'Vomiting gets rid of tension and feelings of panic.'

3 **Over-generalisation:** involves assuming that what is true of a few situations is true of a wide range of other related and unrelated situations.
Examples:
'I was unhappy when I weighed more, so I will be unhappy if my weight increases.'
'When I am thin I am in control of my life.'
'By vomiting I regain control.'

4 **Magnification and minimisation:** involves overestimating or underestimating the significance or value of a particular situation or event.
Examples:
'I feel terrible I have put on two pounds since last week; this is awful.'
'I may have a successful career, but if I can't control my eating I'm worthless.'
'I had a binge at the weekend when I said I wouldn't. I've ruined everything. I'm useless.'

5 **Personalisation:** involves assuming external events have a personal significance when there is little or no evidence that they do.
Examples:
'I'm sure those people noticed how fat I am.'
'I can't eat in front of other people – they will watch me.'
'Everyone hates me.'

6 **Absolutist, dichotomous thinking:** refers to the tendency to place everything in opposite categories. Thinking is extreme and absolute; everything is either black or white, good or bad, right or wrong, all or nothing.
Examples:
'If I'm thin I'm special. If I'm fat I'm disgusting.'
'If I have one more bite I will go completely out of control.'
'I am completely worthless and disgusting for having binged.'

It may be noted that many of the features identified in this list are elaborations of what has been termed the 'anorexic attitude', which as we have seen is crucial in the diagnosis of anorexia and bulimia. If you ask an anorexic why she starves herself, or a bulimic why she binges and purges, you may well receive an answer reflecting some of the 'cognitive distortions' outlined in the above list. The beliefs and assumptions represented here may be regarded as the 'proximal causes' of anorexia and bulimia. While some may want to argue that such ideas predate the onset of the illness, and become exaggerated and entrenched as the illness develops, others would argue these beliefs largely develop as a consequence of the illness and are best regarded as perpetuating or maintaining factors.

Family characteristics. One of the most controversial issues in the area of aetiology is that of family relationships. The claim is often made that family interactions, or dynamics, are crucial aetiological factors. In particular the relationship between the anorexic and her mother has received a great deal of attention. I will treat this in some detail in chapter 4 so will not cover it here.

Socio-cultural factors. Epidemiological studies indicate that between 90 and 95% of anorexic patients are female, the majority are between 14 and 25 years of age, and social classes I and II are over-represented (although the incidence among the other social classes appears to be increasing). While there is evidence of a sharp increase in the incidence of the disorder over the last 50 years among females, the incidence among males has remained static. Also anorexia appears to be largely limited to Western, or 'developed' cultures. It has frequently been claimed that anorexia and bulimia are also largely limited to women of white racial origin. However, recent research in London by psychologist Bridget Dolan, and psychiatrists J. Hubert Lacey and Chris Evans, has found similar levels of disordered eating attitudes and concern with body weight and shape among their samples of white, Afro-Caribbean and Asian women. More work needs to be done in this area but it is suggested that the levels of disturbance identified in women of non-white racial origin is the result of their absorption into Western societies. It appears that being a young woman living in a Western society, whether of white or non-white racial origin, is a major risk factor. Why?

Many writers have drawn attention to particular features of Western societies which may be of aetiological significance. A widely quoted study by David Garner, and his colleagues, looked at the changing standards of female attractiveness over the period 1960 to 1980. The Miss America Pageant and the Playboy Playmate of the Month were taken as their two indices of female attractiveness. They found that over the 20-year period there was a significant shift towards lower weights and less curves (as measured by the width of the hips relative to the waist) for the models in both cases. This general trend was also noticed through an examination of changes in body proportions of fashion models over this period. However, Garner and his colleagues also studied the actual average weights of American women over the same 20-year period and found the reverse trend. While the ideal, or preferred, female body became thinner, the actual average weight of women increased. The authors note that an increase in anorexia nervosa has occurred parallel to both 'our culture's aesthetic preference for thinness in women', and an actual increase in average female body weight.

Of course this study really examined the shift in male preferences. Many questions arise from this, for example, what 'ideal shape' do women have for themselves? Is this dictated by a woman's perception of what is attractive to men?

This and related questions were investigated in 1985 by R. Fallon and P. Rozin, two research psychologists from the University of Pennsylvania. Their subjects were male and female students. The students each examined pictures of males and females of the same height but widely varying weight. Each student was asked to rank the pictures in four ways:

1 The body shape most like their own.
2 The body shape they would most like to have (their 'ideal' weight).
3 The body shape they thought would be most attractive to the opposite sex.
4 The opposite sex body shape that they found most attractive.

It was found that female estimates of their current shape were consistently larger than their actual shape. Their 'ideal' shape was consistently thinner than their actual, or estimated current shape. Interestingly the shape women thought would be most attractive to males was bigger than their own 'ideal shape'. Hence, in this group of young women, their desired, or preferred, body shape was not dictated solely by a desire to be attractive to males.

In contrast to these results the male students average estimates of their current shape, ideal shape, and shape they believed to be most attractive to women, were all consistent. However, on the third series, the male and female results were similar. Both misjudged, but in opposite directions. Females believed males to prefer a thinner female body shape than they actually did, and males believed females to prefer a bigger male body than they actually did.

This, and many other similar studies, have demonstrated that women in our culture experience far greater uncertainty, discontent, discomfort and dissatisfaction with their body shape, than men do with theirs.

Could it be then that pressures to be thin, can contribute to the prevalence of anorexia and bulimia? This hypothesis was tested by David Garner and Paul Garfinkel in Canada, in 1980. They investigated the prevalence of anorexia nervosa among female ballet students and modelling students, and compared these with a group of female university students (pursuing varied studies) and a group of female music students. Ballerinas and models must conform to explicit demands concerning body shape and weight. They experience in an intense form our culture's preference for thinness. If this pressure is a significant factor in the aetiology of anorexia nervosa we should find an increased prevalence of the disorder among such populations. As predicted, Garner and Garfinkel found about 7% of the ballerinas and modelling students met the full diagnostic criteria for anorexia nervosa, although none were currently receiving treatment. This is in the region of ten times the prevalence of anorexia in females of similar age in the general population. As this could be interpreted as the result of achievement and competition pressures, rather than the pressures to be thin, these groups were compared with music students from a prestigious and highly competitive conservatory. None of the women in this group met the diagnostic criteria for anorexia nervosa. Further, the music student's scores on a questionnaire designed to identify eating and weight difficulties (The Eating Attitudes Test), were indistinguishable from those of a group of general university students. This suggests that the emphasis on body weight within the ballerina and modelling populations was the significant factor accounting for the raised prevalence of the disorder. However, Garner and Garfinkel compared the ballet students from a national ballet school to a group of students from a college dance department. It was assumed that the latter group were exposed to similar pressures to be thin, but were in a less competitive environment. They found that the scores on the Eating Attitudes Test were much higher for the ballet students. The authors conclude from this study that it is the combination of pressures to be thin and a highly competitive environment that significantly increased the risk of developing anorexia nervosa.

Hilde Bruch has written extensively of the pressures involved in the 'attempt to fulfil fashion's demands to be skinny'. A slim body shape has become the symbol of success, beauty, competence and worth. The power of slenderness to suggest all that is valued in our culture is evident in the ubiquitous use of a slender body (usually female) to sell anything from shampoo and cars to airline tickets. Psychotherapist Susie Orbach has emphasised the conflict inherent in our 'cultural insistence' that food is the woman's domain (as mother and wife), and that she should strive to maintain a particular shape to attract and provide pleasure for men. A dilemma arises in which women are expected to feed others but not themselves. 'The preoccupation with food is linked with a fetishising of the female form ... Women find themselves obsessively engaged with both their food and their bodies ... Women are constantly engaged in trying to mediate the harrowing effects of culturally induced body insecurity.'

It may be argued that anorexia and bulimia are reflections of the enormous pressures on women to validate their self-worth, and please others, by controlling their appearance. These pressures appear to have been greatly exacerbated by the movement away from traditional family based roles towards the masculine dominated world of careers. Women now have to struggle with the dual expectations of performance and success in the domain of employment, and the demands of physical attractiveness. In terms of aetiology it would seem that some women find these pressures overwhelming. Anorexia and bulimia may be seen as either an extreme act of conformity to such pressures, or an act of rejection and rebellion.

Our model of anorexia and bulimia, as conditions with multiple determinants, suggests the conflicts outlined here may produce stresses which lead to disorders associated with eating and body shape, in women with particular vulnerabilities (perhaps because of the kinds of factors outlined in the sections dealing with individual and family characteristics). Hence these culturally induced conflicts form part of the jigsaw of explanation along with the other factors outlined above. Of course in any individual case the specific constellation of causal factors will be unique, with some factors being more significant than others.

Precipitating factors

A wide range of stressors have been identified which appear to be significant in triggering the decision to lose weight or over-eat. These stressors include: increased achievement pressure (many cases of anorexia nervosa occur just prior to examinations); sexual conflicts or unpleasant sexual experiences, inter-personal conflict, separation or loss (often anorexia is preceded by a family bereavement); distressing pubertal shape changes, the experience of menstruation (which may be felt as an unwanted intrusion, or as further loss of control); an adverse comment about the individual's shape or eating habits; positive remarks about weight loss; comments or reflections to the effect that weight loss is the means to greater control, effectiveness, acceptability, or leverage within the family; socio-economic change, such as loss of income, or promotion, or move to a new location. From the accounts given by bulimics it would appear that the condition can be precipitated by persistent, strong feelings that are experienced as overwhelming or unmanageable. For example, feelings of self-doubt, inferiority, depression, loneliness, anxiety, helplessness and tension, may be significant precipitants of binge eating.

Perpetuating factors

The psychological effects of starvation. Any attempt at explaining anorexic or bulimic behaviour must take account of the effects of starvation. This will of course be most relevant to anorexia but, as has been pointed out in chapter 2, bulimia often involves a very chaotic picture of bingeing and purging alternating with periods of severe food restriction. Although the bulimic does not become emaciated, there will often be considerable fluctuations in body weight. Hence, while this section is of particular relevance to anorexia, it should be borne in mind that this material will also have major implications for bulimia when there are significant periods of food restriction.

It should be noted that anorexia nervosa involves a rather specific form of dietary restriction that has important differences to general starvation. The anorexic typically reduces or eliminates carbohydrate intake, and often restricts food intake to particular types of food, often proteins such as cheese. The anorexic will therefore display characteristics of carbohydrate deprivation rather than features of general starvation. In extreme cases skin colour may be altered by a diet comprised almost entirely of one kind of food, oranges for example.

However research into the effects of general starvation has revealed some very significant information for the study of anorexia and bulimia. The physical effects of starvation have been well known for some time, but we are particularly concerned with how starvation affects the individual psychologically. In a classic study, carried out in the United States during the second world war by A. Keys and his colleagues, 36 volunteers were placed on semi-starvation diets for six months. All participants were psychologically healthy males. The physical and psychological changes occurring in subjects were carefully monitored.

Among the psychological changes noted were:

1 Intense preoccupation with food, cooking and watching others eat. Food became the dominant topic of conversation. Nineteen men began studying cookbooks and collecting recipes. When returning from shopping trips subjects had often purchased cooking or eating utensils which were not needed; subjects were unable to explain such behaviour. Activities centred on the daily food allowance with men spending hours planning how they would eat. Several subjects drew up detailed plans of how they would become chefs.

2 Changes in eating habits included preference for unusual food concoctions, delaying meals, eating extremely slowly, often taking hours to eat what would previously have taken a few minutes.

3 Communication with the men became increasingly difficult, and researchers reported subjects were tending to lie to them.

4 As the study progressed an increase in shoplifting and petty theft was noted. Also hoarding, possessiveness and acquisitiveness, of both food-related items, and items unrelated to food.

5 Subjects became increasingly self-centred, hostile, withdrawn and antisocial.
6 Loss of sexual interest was noted in the decline in reports of sexual fantasies, dreams, and masturbation.
7 Episodes of uncontrolled eating (bingeing) followed by vomiting were recorded. Subjects reported intense feelings of guilt and self-disgust after such episodes.
8 Drinking tea, coffee, water, chewing of gum, smoking and nail-biting all substantially increased.
9 Sleep disturbance, restlessness and agitation were common.
10 Emotional changes included recurring bouts of depression, accompanied by low self-esteem, intense self-criticism, guilt, and self-hatred.
11 Substantial increases in a range of 'neurotic' traits were noted, including increased anxiety, hypochondriasis, hysteria, and obsessionality.
12 Pronounced fluctuations in mood were also recorded, with one subject requiring hospitalisation for treatment of hypomania.
13 The subjects showed severe restrictions in conceptual ability. Polarisation of thinking, reducing ideas to simple black and white terms, was very common.
14 Difficulties in concentration, alertness, and even ambition were also recorded.

The researchers involved in this study have stressed that individuals varied considerably in the extent to which starvation altered their behaviour and personality. With some of the volunteers the changes were so profound that they were withdrawn from the study. It is also important to note that for many of the subjects the psychological changes did not disappear once normal eating and weight had been re-established. In many cases disturbance persisted for three months or more after the study had ended and normal eating had begun. Also many of the subjects found 're-feeding' extremely unpleasant and stressful. Many reported being confused and anxious about the way their body responded to eating (for example in feeling extremely hungry after a large meal).

Although there are obvious differences between the experiences of these volunteers and that of anorexics, this study clearly has important implications for our understanding of the origin of many of the symptoms of anorexia. Also, in cases where bingeing and purging alternate with starvation, there are significant implications for our understanding of bulimia.

For example, the bulimic may use periods of starvation as a form of purging. However, the food restriction actually creates the conditions in which the next binge is made more likely. As the study has shown, deprived of food an individual becomes preoccupied with eating and in this condition some will binge at the first opportunity. Hence where starvation follows bingeing, the food restrictions, rather than working to counteract the binge, actually perpetuate the cycle. In the section on predisposing factors it was noted that personality can change profoundly as a result of starvation. The study by Keys and his colleagues provides a powerful demonstration of this. It seems clear that certain characteristic features of anorexia and bulimia may be attributed directly to the effects of starvation. But starvation on its own cannot account for all of the features of these conditions. Typically the anorexic is not disturbed by her condition. The state of starvation is highly valued, in some way it is experienced as rewarding.

Forms of reinforcement. A vast body of experimental work demonstrates that behaviours which are followed by some kind of reward will continue to occur (in which case we say the behaviours have been 'positively reinforced'), while behaviours with negative consequences will tend not to occur (a process termed 'aversive conditioning'). Also some behaviours are rewarded in that they stop unpleasant experiences (we say of these behaviours that they have been 'negatively reinforced'). There have been many suggestions offered to explain how weight loss, bingeing and purging, may be rewarded, or reinforced. What links many of these suggestions is the idea that in some way anorexia or bulimia offers a solution to intrapersonal, or interpersonal, problems. For example, where achievement demands are an important precipitant of weight loss, a subsequent relaxation of pressure to achieve may provide a powerful reward for weight loss (in this case we would say weight loss has been 'negatively reinforced'). Similarly we have noted that Western culture associates personal success, control, and worth, with dietary restraint and a slender figure. This association may be accepted in an exaggerated form by the anorexic so that her sense of personal effectiveness or self-worth, becomes intrinsically tied to her ability to control her weight. With such associations being thin becomes 'positively reinforced'. In addition, as weight increase comes to represent failure, it becomes highly aversive, and hence weight loss is highly reinforced.

Hilde Bruch has argued that at the heart of the anorexic syndrome is a 'paralysing sense of ineffectiveness', where the issue of control is crucial. If this is correct then the control of weight may be one area in which the individual feels some measure of effectiveness or autonomy. In this case her dietary behaviour may serve to counter other feelings of loss of control, dependence and ineffectiveness. Once again weight loss becomes highly reinforced as it leads to a sense of control or mastery, and weight increase becomes very aversive because it is associated with loss of control. Many anorexics come to experience a sense of self-identity through their 'special' thinness. 'Giving up' anorexia and putting on weight can be experienced as a threat to self, and a loss of uniqueness and individuality.

A powerful form of reinforcement that appears to be significant for many women with bulimia is the maintenance of sexual attractiveness. Heavier body weight is associated with rejection and dislike, whereas slimness is associated with receiving attention and sexual desirability. A more obvious form of reinforcement occurs in bulimia where the attempt to control eating creates a very unpleasant state of tension, letting go and eating may be experienced as a relief, or the release from tension may occur through vomiting. Bingeing often acts like an anaesthetic and blocks out unwanted feelings. Similarly after the binge feelings of depression, guilt, panic and discomfort may be reduced by vomiting. Hence in various ways bingeing and vomiting may be experienced as rewarding, it actually does work as a way of getting rid of unwanted feelings – at least temporarily. Another powerful form of reinforcement may involve the function that an eating disorder comes to have in the family, we will consider this in the next chapter.

Two accounts of the reinforcing nature of starvation have been particularly influential. We saw in the section on predisposing factors that some people may, for various reason, be ill equipped to deal with the adjustment demands associated with puberty. Although they may not be aware of the reason for their anxieties, such individuals may experience low body weight, with the accompanying suppression of sexual development, a considerable relief. Hence for such people starvation or low body weight will be reinforced, and weight increase will then become aversive. As we have seen, Professor Crisp has developed these ideas in some detail, regarding the anorexic condition to be a form of 'psychobiological regression', involving a phobic response to post-pubertal body weight. In this view anorexia is maintained by the fact that the feared maturational crisis is avoided when the individual remains at low body weight.

A second account involves the claim that the effects of starvation are significant in that they are progressive (i.e. they come to influence the total range of experience), and they are addictive. Psychotherapist Marilyn Duker and psychologist Roger Slade have presented an account along these lines which they refer to as the 'whirlpool theory of starvation', which they contrast to the 'psychobiological regression' theory mentioned in the previous paragraph.

Duker and Slade note 'starvation plays a crucial part in creating the symptoms of anorexia nervosa', and that starvation 'create(s) most of the incomprehensible behaviour', associated with the condition. They liken the effects of starvation to a whirlpool. Someone may begin to control their food intake, and lose weight, for a variety of reasons, but as weight falls thinking becomes progressively more polarised, and simplified. The classic 'anorexic attitude' becomes stronger and embraces an ever wider range of issues; that is, the individual's entire life comes under the dominance of the fat equals bad, thin equals good polarisation. Just as a whirlpool accelerates as it spirals into its centre, so too, as weight falls, the psychological change accelerates. On the outer edges of the whirlpool it is relatively easy to see alternative courses of action and to avoid the spiral by 'getting off', so to speak. But as you move from the outer edges to the inner region of the spiral the easiest option is to continue on the spiral. Going back, or 'getting off', becomes increasingly difficult, as you continue to spiral into the centre. Hence, at different parts of the spiral, or at different stages of starvation, there may be different reasons for continuing, but gradually choice and genuine decision-making become severely restricted. In many ways this process resembles the development of an addiction. Anorexics often report feelings of well-being which appear to be related to an increased sense of effectiveness and control, decisiveness and a reduction in powerful emotions, similar to the effects of certain classes of addictive drugs. This positive effect is in contrast to the effects noted in the study by Keys described above. The positive experience appears to be due in part to the physiological changes, but to a greater extent results from the simplification and polarisation of thinking being experienced as pleasurable to the anorexic in contrast to the inner turmoil and distress associated with heavier weights. It would seem then that a person gets drawn into the whirlpool of starvation because certain features of starvation offer a firmer sense of self-identity and wellbeing than that experienced at normal weight.

To summarise: the 'psychobiological regression' theory sees a major factor in the maintenance of anorexia as being specifically the avoidance of sexual maturity with its accompanying challenge to identity and sense of self. The 'whirlpool theory' offers a more complex account which sees the special effects of starvation as being reinforcing in that the individual gets drawn into, and 'hooked' on, the sense of control, effectiveness and identity experienced at low weight. What unites these two theories is that whatever prompted dieting to begin with, and there may be many reasons, the state of starvation is experienced as rewarding. In some way it offers a resolution of conflicts centering on issues of self-identity.

There are many ways in which starvation, or bingeing and vomiting, are rewarded or reinforced, but it may be objected that surely the long-term consequences of these behaviours are highly negative, even destructive; hence should the behaviours not cease? That is, should they not be eliminated by the proess of 'aversive conditioning'? Research into the way in which the consequences of specific behaviour determine the likelihood of that behaviour being repeated (i.e. the study of 'operant conditioning') has demonstrated that one crucial variable is time. Generally speaking consequences that immediately follow from a behaviour will tend to have a greater impact in terms of increasing (through positive effects) or decreasing (through negative effects) the likelihood of the behaviour being repeated, than consequences that follow some time later. Generally speaking short-term consequences have greater power to influence behaviour than long-term consequences. This simple principle offers a very useful explanation for a very wide range of puzzling behaviours. In the context of anorexia and bulimia the immediate reinforcement from feeling a sense of control and identity, or release from tension, often override the long-term problems associated with poor physical health, low self-esteem and other psychological difficulties.

Summary

This chapter has presented a model of anorexia and bulimia as conditions with multiple determinants. It appears that a range of factors, including individual, family, and cultural characteristics, contribute to the development of eating disorders. Similarly we can identify various events which may 'trigger' the condition in those with specific vulnerabilities. Once developed, powerful forces inherent in the condition itself serve to maintain the disorder. However, despite the complex aetiological picture which has emerged from various lines of research, one view about the causes of anorexia and bulimia has been widely held for many years. This is the claim that ultimately parents are to blame for their daughter's condition. We will examine this claim in the next chapter.

4 Are parents to blame?

In his classic account of anorexia nervosa, Lasègue, writing in 1873, noted: 'This description ... would be incomplete without reference to their homelife. Both the patient and her family form a tightly knit whole, and we obtain a false picture of the disease if we limit our observation to the patient alone.' More pointedly, an account written 200 years ago (1789) by the French physician J. Naudeau suggested an anorexic's death was due to the influence of her mother.

William Gull, who we have noted introduced the term 'anorexia nervosa', urged that for treatment to be successful patients should be separated from their families. Other early accounts have described a tendency for parents of anorexics to be disturbed themselves, and a tendency for hospitalised anorexics to deteriorate when visited by their mothers.

The claim that parents of anorexics have specific attitudes, behaviours, and patterns of interaction, which somehow induce illness in their daughters, is encountered very frequently in the literature on eating disorders. This view, that in some way parents (especially mothers) are responsible for their daughter's illness, has permeated lay and professional opinion alike.

Case example
A mother of a 14-year-old anorexic visited her daughter in hospital. She found staff very uncommunicative about her daughter's treatment. One of the nurses suggested she should not visit her daughter for a while. After her daughter was discharged from hospital this mother recalled her experience with considerable distress: 'I know you people say its all the parents' fault, but we've tried our best. All we've ever wanted was for her to be well and happy. Just tell us what to do to help. We don't want to be told that our daughter is better off without us; we've loved and cared for her all her life. But the way the doctor and nurses looked at us when we visited ... I knew what they were thinking. As if we had made her ill, and had no right

to know what was going to happen to her. They wouldn't tell us anything. We desperately wanted help for her, and were relieved when she went into hospital. But they made us feel as if we had no idea how to treat our daughter. They seemed to think they cared for her more than us. Can they really believe that? Don't they understand she's our daughter? Do they know what that means?'

The experience of this mother is by no means unusual. The tendency to blame parents for their daughter's condition is clearly presented in a book by Peter Lambley called *How to Survive Anorexia*. Lambley, a GP, claims that 'parents of anorexics were capable of a high degree of cruelty and disinterest'. Needless to say such claims are a source of considerable distress for parents. When working in this field one frequently encounters parents who have taken these claims very seriously and have added a burden of guilt to the anxiety they already experience for their daughter's safety. But what is the evidence for these claims? Are parents really to blame? In this chapter we will look at some of the more influential accounts of the family context of anorexia and return to answer this question at the end. When people claim 'parents' cause anorexia they usually mean 'mothers'; we will start with the most influential account of the mother-daughter relationship.

'Anorexogenic mothers'?

In chapter 3 we considered individual and cultural factors which may predispose an individual to develop anorexia or bulimia. It was noted that, although at one level the distinction between the individual, family, and culture are obvious, in terms of our study of factors contributing to a vulnerability to develop anorexia or bulimia these distinctions become blurred. Individual and cultural factors meet in the family; the family forms both the context of individual development and the mediator of cultural values.

As we have seen, Hilde Bruch considers developmental problems which underlie anorexia nervosa to arise in the context of a particular form of mother-child relationship. Briefly, Bruch suggests that these mothers are over-anxious and preoccupied with their child's well-being. Such mothers are extremely

conscientious and efficient at providing and caring for their in-
fants. This may occur for many reasons, but could lead to an 'over-
valuing' of the child together with high expectations. This over-
anxious and at times self-sacrificing attitude leads the mother
to persistently anticipate the child's needs. This tendency may
manifest in the earliest stages of the child's life around feeding
and physical needs. For example food is given promptly before
strong feelings of hunger are experienced. This may result in a
disturbance in the child's ability to differentiate her own needs
from what are external influences. Because mother habitually
indicates what should be her daughter's needs, what becomes
important or real is what other people say she feels. This
developmental context, along with the specific developmental
problems noted in chapter 3, produce serious difficulties in the
area of personal autonomy. That is, as the child develops, her
demands for independence clash with her early conditioning
that mother 'knows best'. Often anorexics report feeling they
have been living someone else's life, and that in some way
control of weight and food intake was the only way to gain some
measure of personal worth, autonomy and control. In Bruch's
account, and in similar descriptions which draw on her work,
the claim is made that certain features of the mother-daughter
relationship can lead to developmental problems which may
contribute to the development of anorexia or bulimia. It is from
such accounts that the claim that it is the mother's behaviour
that leads to anorexia (that is, that some mothers are
'anorexogenic') derives support. We will consider the difficulties
associated with proving this claim at the end of the next section.

'Anorexic families'?

Some writers have focused on the family as a unit rather than
the early mother-child relationship. Arthur Crisp, for example,
although rejecting the idea that there is a single family type
associated with anorexia, has suggested that certain family
constellations may inhibit, or even prohibit, adolescent maturation in children, thus providing a context in which maturation
will present severe adjustment problems.

But the most elaborate descriptions of families with an anorexic member have been provided by Maria Selvini Palazolli,

and Salvadore Minuchin. Palazolli has worked extensively with families of anorexics in Milan, Italy. She has focused on the 'anorexogenic' features of families; that is, the sorts of characteristics believed to produce anorexia. Minuchin working in Philadelphia in the USA, has investigated the families of people with a range of 'psychosomatic' symptoms (e.g. gastrointestinal disorders). In his studies of the families of anorexics he considers the entire family to be 'symptomatic', not just the individual. Hence he would consider the family as a whole to be anorexic. We will look at these views in turn.

Palazolli and Minuchin present 'systems models' of families with an anorexic member. This type of model considers each member of the system to be both a causal agent in themselves, and as being the recipient of causal influences from other members of the system. Because the family as a system is a uniquely interlocking and interdependent whole, analysis of individuals in isolation will inevitably be inadequate. Both writers claim it is possible to identify specific characteristics of families with an anorexic member, and that these family contexts, or systems, create and sustain the symptoms of anorexia.

Palazolli emphasises the following characteristics:

1 **Lack of conflict resolution.** These families present an image of harmony which in fact conceals deep resentments and bitterness. Often there are profound disappointments and hostilities. These conflicts remain concealed beneath a facade of unity and politeness, they are never openly acknowledged or addressed.

2 **Marital disillusionment.** Beneath a superficial pleasantness and display of unity the marital relationship is characterised by profound disappointment. This sense of disillusionment can take many forms, frequently centering on career, status, or sexual issues. But regardless of the particular source of the disappointment, the essential factor is that these feelings remain hidden. These unacknowledged feelings of disappointment and disillusionment profoundly alter the relationships and interactions within the family.

3 **Self-sacrifice.** The marital disillusionment is dealt with partly by each partner striving to demonstrate their 'moral superiority' by making sacrifices for the family. Hilde Bruch outlines a similar feature in her descriptions of families with an anorexic member.

4 **Covert coalitions.** Overt alliancies between parent and child are not permitted, but beneath the appearance of harmony the child forms secret alliances with each parent. Through these

alliances parents seek some relief from personal disappointment, and the child comes to play a central role in holding the family together and keeping conflicts hidden. Palazolli calls this 'three way matrimony'.

Minuchin presents a similar list of characteristics, although he claims these features are not unique to anorexia, rather they describe any family in which a member has some form of 'psychosomatic' problem. Minuchin identifies the following characteristics:

1 **Enmeshment.** Family members are over-involved with one another. Privacy is not respected, and is likely to be regarded with suspicion, as evidence of disloyalty. Family members intrude on each other's thoughts and feelings which become, as it were, family property. Independence, autonomy, separation, and individual identity, are difficult issues for such families. Minuchin also describes parents showing an intrusive interest in their daughter's physical development. Changes in body shape, menstruation, etc., are somehow parental property. As a result of this enmeshed state the daughter does not experience her development and what is happening in her body as 'hers'.

2 **Over-protectiveness.** Members are over-concerned with each other's welfare. Parents observe their children's behaviour in minute detail and strive to guide them through careful scrutiny and imposition of family rules. Wide-ranging parental control is exercised under the pretext of love and concern, making it very difficult for the child to rebel without immense guilt. The child monitors her behaviour and her parents responses carefully, and strives to conform so as to avoid the guilt and threat of independence. The child is controlled and imposed upon 'for her own good'. Although this over-protectiveness serves the parent's needs rather than the child's, this fact is disowned. Family members are adept at denying their own needs overtly while covertly expressing their deeper or inner wishes. This feature is very close to the spirit of self-sacrifice described by Palazolli and Bruch.

3 **Rigidity.** Families are highly resistant to change, hence the onset of adolescence in a child is likely to be met with attempts to keep the individual as a child. Childish responses will be met with approval (perhaps with statements like: 'That's my little girl'), while displays of independence, autonomy, sexuality, and power, will be punished, often through emotional blackmail (reflected in statements such as: 'What have we done to deserve this; you're not my little girl').

4 **Avoidance of conflict.** Open expression of conflict is a family taboo. Conflict may simply be denied, or allowed only over trivial issues. Or there may be a pattern of confrontation on the part of one of the parents, while the other functions as a diffuser. Either way conflicts go underground while a picture of harmony is created on the surface. This characteristic is also discussed at length by Palazolli.

Minuchin regards the key factor in the development and maintenance of symptoms to be the child's involvement in parental conflict. Palazolli also describes symptoms in terms of their function in the family. Although there may be different patterns of involvement, the essential point is that the child, rather than conflict between the parents, becomes the family problem. This focus on the child's symptoms serves to express as well as avoid the unresolved conflicts existing between the parents. Palazolli offers a similar account of the functional role of anorexic symptoms in which she sees the child as a mediator of parental conflict.

Minuchin and Palazolli claim that the demands of adolescence, involving issues of independence, autonomy, self-identity, etc., are especially threatening to children who have grown up in such families.

But what evidence is there that these families really do give rise to anorexia? It is important to note that when reading the literature in this area one is immediately struck by the inadequacy of the evidence. It is important to acknowledge the serious deficiencies of research in this area, because sympathy for the very real suffering involved in these disorders can lead one to look for scapegoats. That is, parents can become a focus for the difficult feelings anorexic women arouse in others.

The first difficulty is the same as that noted in the section on personality characteristics. Most studies are retrospective, hence we cannot determine the sorts of features the family had before the illness developed. To simply describe the conflicts and difficulties of families with an anorexic member is not to elucidate factors relevant to the origin of the illness, because it would be very surprising to find a family in which one member is systematically starving themselves to be a model of harmony. The illness itself will affect the family in complex ways and without reliable data on the family before the illness developed we cannot assume post-illness characteristics provide evidence for the origin of the disorder. A second major problem is that most, if not all, studies lack adequate controls. That is, we are not able to make reliable comparisons between families with an anorexic member and families without. Can we really be sure the family conflicts described in the literature are significantly associated with anorexia? How do these families compare with non-anorexic, families? Would we expect any family with an adolescent daughter to be free of conflict? What are families like where daughters have other problems, say drug abuse? or a physical disability? These comparisons have not been made. Most of the information on 'anorexic families' is of an anecdotal nature, often based on a single case, which may be useful in generating hypotheses but are not adequate substitutes for controlled research.

Certainly most workers in this field would reject the idea that there is one particular family pattern, such as a dominant mother, involved in the development of anorexia. The evidence, such as it is at present, suggests that families with an anorexic daughter may show certain characteristics. It is impossible at present to say how significant these similarities are in terms of aetiology. Further, from the multi-dimensional perspective adopted in this book, the strongest claim we could make would be that family characteristics may turn out to be of aetiological significance among a range of other factors. Given the model outlined in chapter 3, family characteristics may contribute to the development of the disorder but could not be regarded as 'the cause' of the condition. It may turn out to be more accurate to regard family context as a perpetuating rather than predisposing factor. At the moment we do not know.

The family as bearer of culture

In chapter 3 we considered various socio-cultural factors which may be significant in predisposing individuals to develop anorexia or bulimia. The family is the mediator between the growing child and society. The family initiates and adapts the child into their culture. It has been argued that certain families amplify the sorts of cultural characteristics which we have noted may predispose to anorexia or bulimia. For example, consider our cultural obsession with physical appearance, shape and weight. The question arises: Do we find a greater preoccupation with these issues in families with an anorexic or bulimic member than families without?

There are many anecdotal reports of a high prevalence of weight control, obesity, vegetarians, special dieting needs, exercise, and preoccupation with appearance, on the part of parents with an anorexic or bulimic family member. However, evidence from adequately controlled research is very slender. The most clear-cut finding appears to be that of an unusually high prevalence of maternal obesity in families with a bulimic anorexic.

Palazolli and Bruch, in particular, have emphasised the changing role of women in Western societies, and the specific stresses that this change has produced. Some families may reproduce these tensions in an acute form. For example, some families may be preoccupied with achievement and success and put immense pressure on their children to do well academically, or pursue particular careers. To this may be added the further pressure to behave in a traditionally 'feminine' way. A traditional female role stereotype, i.e. being nurturing, feeding others, being passive, etc., clashes with the values of a striving, acquisitive society, which encourages people to 'get on'. This conflict can be amplified in family life, producing intolerable stresses.

Another perspective considers anorexogenic, or anorexic, families to be microcosms of a patriarchal society. Hence, it is argued, the position of females in such families is characteristic of the position of women in societies dominated by male power. In a sense such families have resisted movements towards the emancipation of women in society at large, and represent forces of patriarchy opposed to change. As clinical psychologist Gill Edwards has noted: 'From this viewpoint anorexia may be seen not so much as the result of pathogenic families but as an almost inevitable consequence of the clash between continuing patriarchy are our supposedly 'liberated', 'egalitarian' society.' The descriptions of anorexogenic, or anorexic, families given by Palazolli and Minuchin can certainly be seen as 'patriarchal', rather than 'egalitarian'. For example, the intolerance of change, rebellion, autonomy, or independence, and the intrusive, controlling concern with the child's functioning, does seem to reflect the oppressive attitude to women characteristic of a patriarchal system. On the basis of these views anorexia may be regarded as an act of protest against gender expectations, in which a woman is using the only weapon at her disposal: her body. However, as writer Kim Chernin has suggested, it may be argued that anorexia is an act of conformity in which the anorexic becomes a non-threatening, submissive child in order to please 'the patriarchy'.

As we have seen, theories which focus on the family as a system tend to view the symptoms of anorexia or bulimia as operating functionally within the system. Views which emphasise the socialising function of families stress the way in which the family mediates social or cultural values, in particular as regards the role of women. This material has been drawn from some of the more influential writers who have contributed to this debate. In the following section I will outline some anecdotal observations on the family context of anorexia and bulimia from my own clinical practice.

Anecdotes and clinical impressions

The idea that parents or families in some way cause anorexia or bulimia has been presented in a number of forms. Some writers focus on the relationship between mother and daughter; and indeed when people say parents cause anorexia or bulimia they usually mean mothers. Other writers have considered the wider network of relationships within the family. Some writers have argued certain types of mother-daughter relationship, or certain types of family, may predispose an individual to develop an eating disorder. Others focus on the family as a context in which anorexic or bulimic symptoms are maintained.

I have already commented on the lack of controlled research in this area. However, it is an undeniable fact that the view that families, in particular mothers, are crucial factors in understanding the origin of eating disorders, has been an enormously influential and extremely persistent idea. Despite the lack of adequate research many clinicians have commented on the significance of the anorexic daughter's relationship to her mother. In her book *The Anorexic Experience* psychotherapist Marilyn Lawrence notes: 'I can say with certainty that I have never worked with an anorexic woman who has a 'straightforward' relationship with her mother.' Lawrence emphasises that this does not mean that anorexics have a bad relationship with their mothers, but rather that 'the relationships are normally complex and puzzling to both mother and daughter.' Their relationship may well seem complex and puzzling to the anorexic and her mother, but it is surprising how often outsiders imagine the whole situation can be summed up in a very simple formula. The idea that the relationship between a mother and her anorexic daughter is somehow involved in the production or maintenance of the anorexic symptoms is a very compelling one because feeding is such an essential part of 'mothering'. Feeding is easily equated with caring; giving food is giving love. It is a simple step to say rejection of food is a rejection of love. This simple equation, refusing to eat equals rejection of mother's love, is one that is often suggested as an explanation for what is happening between the anorexic and her mother. But, in my experience, the situation is never that simple.

'We're very close. Mother's the only person who understands me.' Anorexics often make such statements. I have also been struck by the number of times symptoms of anorexia occur before major life events such as examinations, or going away to university, or starting a career. The stresses of such situations may involve conflicts surrounding achievement, but the difficulties of these situations are often described by anorexics in terms of separation. That is, such events herald leaving home, and specifically leaving mother. In such situations the desire for independence, separation, and autonomy, may conflict with a desire for nurturance, safety, and closeness. Given this conflict the anorexic's feelings towards her mother are unlikely to be 'straightforward'. However, it should also be borne in mind that separation will evoke powerful feelings in the mother. The potential separation and the evident distress and incapacity of her daughter will inevitably lead to difficult emotions that must be dealt with, in most cases, without understanding or help from anyone else.

Marilyn Lawrence observes that the relationship between the anorexic and her mother is often characterised by 'ambivalence' (the experience of very positive and very negative feelings towards the same person), and by difficulties about separateness and differentiation. My own experience would confirm this observation. After a brief discussion in which mother is idealised anorexics will often express feelings of disappointment or resentment towards their mothers. Similarly many mothers express conflicting feelings towards their daughters, for example, protectiveness and resentment. The negative feelings often cause a great deal of distress and even guilt. Now it is often noted that ambivalence is a common characteristic of relationships between mothers and their daughters in our society, it is certainly not unique to anorexics and their mothers. Although this may be the case it should be noted that the tensions associated with ambivalent feelings become greatly amplified in the context of anorexia nervosa, where guilt and self-criticism on the part of the anorexic and her mother are such prominent features.

Although the relationship between anorexic daughters and their fathers has received relatively little attention, fathers are clearly of great importance in the life of the sufferer. It appears that fathers with anorexic daughters are often 'over-involved' in the sense that they have played an unusually active part in the upbringing of their daughter perhaps because of spending long periods of time at home through illness or having specific career expectations which are constantly kept before the growing child. The other situation frequently encountered is where father is disengaged and distant. These fathers tend to regard bringing up children to be the mothers domain. Often these fathers remain involved while the family functions smoothly, and perhaps early in their daughter's life were over-involved, but disengage if there are problems that cannot be dealt with by an authoritarian approach (in which the basic message is 'eat this or else'). My own contact with such 'disengaged' fathers has, in every case, revealed someone who is extremely distressed and anxious about their daughter's illness but is paralysed by it. Such fathers typically deal with any powerful feelings by withdrawing and focusing their attention on something else. Their disengagement from their daughter is part of a much more general difficulty of coping with feelings. (This of course is not an uncommon characteristic of males in our culture.)

In describing mother-daughter and father-daughter relationships on this anecdotal level, we may identify characteristics frequently encountered in families with an anorexic member. But it should be remembered that there is no evidence that there is a specific (i.e. unique) pattern of dysfunction in an anorexic's family relationships, or that families 'cause' anorexia or bulimia. The point being made here is that there are often complex relationship problems between anorexic daughters and their mothers and fathers, and that these problems are part of a network of difficulties that may influence the course of the ill-ness. These problems often seem to involve conflicting desires. On the one hand there is a desire for separation, independence and autonomy, on the other hand there is a desire for safety, warmth, nurturance. These are issues not only for the anorexic but also for her mother and father. These conflicts are not unique to families with an anorexic member, in fact this very conflict is a common part of normal adolescent development.

The anorexic becomes terrified of weight gain. It may be argued weight comes to represent (literally and symbolically) maturity, independence, autonomy, and separation. But fear is not the monopoly of the anorexic. Parents often experience their anorexic daughter as an extremely powerful destructive force within the family. It is not unusual for anorexia to dominate family routines, not just in the area of food but also in areas such as how loud the TV is, who is invited to the house, who the family will and will not visit, and how high the heating should be. One mother described how her life had become an endless struggle to avoid upsetting her daughter: 'It's like being on a knife edge. I'm always thinking: how can I get her to eat without provoking a tantrum. If I put too much on her plate she explodes, and says I'm always 'picking on her'. She gets so furious, I'm afraid she will kill herself when she's like that.' This mother also described the 'impossibility' of having a genuine conversation with her daughter. If she said her daughter looked better, her daughter interprets this as meaning she looks fat, and she will stop eating for a few days. The distortions in thinking which occur, or get magnified, with starvation can present severe difficulties in communication.

In this section I have been outlining observations of an anecdotal nature. In my own work with anorexics and bulimics and their families my 'clinical impression' has been that where difficulties in family relationships appear to be inhibiting recovery the problems centre on two main issues: first, the level of over-involvement; second, how the family deals with emotions.

I am not suggesting that all families of anorexics or bulimics have these characteristics, or indeed that such features are unique to these families. Whether these features were present before the eating disorder developed, or whether they arose in response to the illness, I do not know. But it does seem that these two characteristics are often present, and when they are they have a crucial impact on the course of the disorder. This is probably related to the fact that anorexia and bulimia are so intimately related to problems of establishing a sense of self-identity, and self-esteem, and a sense of personal control and effectiveness. Hence I have frequently found that the two issues have to be addressed if recovery is to occur.

Concerning the first part, the level of over-involvement, Minuchin as we have seen noted this feature in his work with families and termed it 'enmeshment'. Being over-involved will often manifest as a lack of clear boundaries between family members. This can take many forms, but often results in lack of respect for privacy. Hence, parents may read their daughter's diaries, or open their letters, or enter their room without knocking. Parents may give a strong message that they have a right to know everything their daughter is doing or thinking. This intrusion can lead to profound feelings of violation and lack of control. Through this behaviour parents may plunge their daughter into a secret world of her own where she will try to create some private space in order to experience some level of control and have some sense of autonomy.

Related to this is a tendency for parents to 'infantilise' their daughter. I have often heard fathers refer to their anorexic daughter as 'my little girl', even when she is in her twenties. In such cases it appears that the parents are finding it difficult to adjust to what amounts to the loss of a young child, and hence they try to preserve a relationship which may have been appropriate to a small child but is certainly not to a young woman. Once again it is important to point out that such a relationship often involves the daughter 'playing the part' of a young girl. There seems to be a profound conflict of desires, as noted above, in which growth, maturity, independence, are both desired and feared, and the protection and security of home is wanted but also deeply resented. Often the presence of an eating disorder provokes even greater over-involvement as parents may try to control their daughter's eating.

Concerning the second area, dealing with emotions, families

may strive to present an image of closeness and normality, and be very concerned that family members are nice to each other and get on well with each other. This can lead to a tendency to deny conflict in the family, and because conflict is usually ignored the family does not develop effective methods of resolving disagreement (as noted poor conflict resolution is a feature identified by both Pallazoli and Minuchin). Because such families believe conflict or arguments should not occur between family members, the idea that disagreements can be healthy, and especially the idea that teenage rebellion is healthy and perhaps even necessary, is extremely unpalatable. Anger is typically denied or dealt with very poorly. Family members experience a great deal of pressure to be nice to each other, to like each other, and to agree with each other. Differences are discouraged, as they may lead to conflict. Major arguments are invariably seen as a disaster. This taboo on hostile feelings extends to self-assertion, which is also seen as selfish and disruptive.

However, it is not merely anger that is seen as threatening, and therefore avoided, other feelings are also strongly denied. Sexual feelings for example may be denied and discouraged. Signs of developing sexual interest may not be accepted by parents as healthy and natural but responded to with anxiety, as if it were a threat. Onset of menstruation may be greeted with embarrassment, reproach, even pity.

A wide range of emotional experience and expression may be denied, or considered too disruptive. Related to this is a tendency for parents to attribute feelings to their daughter that they would prefer her to have, rather than allowing her to experience and express what she actually feels. The tendency to attribute feelings to a child when she doesn't in fact experience those feelings may undermine a developing sense of self-identity, and her ability to manage potentially disruptive feelings such as anger. Anorexics and bulimics often describe experiencing a profound split in how they behave in front of others, especially family members, and what is occurring inside. They feel themselves continuously observed and judged by others with little real permission to explore, express themselves, or grow.

Are parents to blame?

It is both profoundly mistaken and profoundly unjust to blame parents for their daughter's anorexia or bulimia. The current body of research evidence strongly supports the claim that anorexia and bulimia are 'multi-determined'. That is, they result from the specific interaction and timing of a wide range of contributory factors. Now it has been suggested that families may be one factor among others, predisposing an individual to develop an eating disorder. Also the family may be the context of a precipitating stress of some kind, and may also be crucial in perpetuating the disorder. The research evidence for this claim is actually very slender. But let us assume it is true. Does it follow that parents are to blame? Assuming particular family relationships play a part in the aetiology of anorexia and bulimia does not provide any grounds for blame. It is essential to make a clear distinction between the concept of 'cause' and the concept of 'blame'.

Imagine a mother feeding her infant with milk. She is very proud of her daughter, very happy and eager to take care of all her needs. However, unknown to the mother the milk she feeds the infant is contaminated with bacteria. The infant becomes ill. What is the cause of the illness?

> The bacteria?
> Government health policy?
> The manufacturers of the milk?
> The mother for feeding the baby?
> The baby for drinking?
> The milkman for delivering the milk?
> The farmer?

All of the factors listed played a part. The illness resulted from a number of contributory causes. Now we could look at this example in more detail to classify the causes and assess their significance but the question I want to emphasise is this: Who should we blame for the infant's illness? In this case the mother may well blame herself, but would you blame her? Most people would probably accept that while the mother actually played a part in the sequence of events that led to the illness it would be very unjust to blame her for it and quite preposterous to say she didn't care for her child. Blame seems appropriate when someone deliberately causes something bad to occur, or if they neglect a responsibility to prevent something bad occurring. In both cases knowledge of consequences would seem to be necessary before we can, in justice, apportion blame.

I hope this does not sound like a mere verbal quibble. If it is true that in some cases of anorexia and bulimia aspects of family relationships have contributed to the development of the illness, we may be justified in talking about the role of families as contributory 'causes' of anorexia and bulimia, but we are not thereby justified in blaming families.

Assigning cause is not the same as assigning blame. If we think, speak, or act as if they were we are not only seriously mistaken, we are also committing a serious injustice.

Summary

We have considered various descriptions of the families of anorexics and bulimics, and various ways in which it has been argued the family may contribute either to predisposing or perpetuating anorexia and bulimia. Much of this work is speculative and anecdotal. However, it is clearly unavoidable that family relationships will be of major significance in the development and course of such disruptive problems as anorexia and bulimia. I have argued that is is both mistaken and unjust to adopt an attitude of blame towards families, which in particular means mothers. Whatever processes occur within the family it is clear that in the vast majority of cases families do all they can to help the anorexic or bulimic member. The next two chapters will consider the problems facing families with an anorexic or bulimic member, and the ways in which parents, relatives and friends can help the process of recovery.

5 How can parents help?

The question that is the topic of this chapter is one I have been asked very many times by the parents of anorexics and bulimics I have worked with in therapy. It must be stressed at the outset that each situation is unique, and there can be no hard and fast rules that will ensure parents 'do the right thing'. The relationship between parents and their anorexic or bulimic daughter is often a complex mix of dependence and desire for autonomy on the daughter's side, and anger, anxiety and guilt on the parent's side. Occasionally one of the parents will withdraw completely. In chapter 4 I have stressed the futility of seeking to apportion blame, and recommend the far more constructive attitude of concentrating on what can be done to prevent the exacerbation and perpetuation of the problem. It is clear that parents, and the other family members, can do a great deal to help the process of recovery. This principle should be borne in mind by all those involved with the sufferer: the important thing is to provide help and understanding, not to apportion blame.

The first point to take note of is that different forms of help will be required at different stages in the development of anorexia or bulimia. The question then becomes: 'What type of help and when?' A useful framework for answering this question is to think in terms of the three stages of anorexia outlined by Peter Slade, a clinical psychologist in Liverpool. The three stages are:

1 An early stage during which the anorexic discovers that a degree of satisfaction and self-worth can be obtained through weight control, hence she enthusiastically pursues weight control through dieting and possibly exercise.
2 A second stage when the pursuit of thinness becomes relentless, weight control becomes the central organising principle of her life, and her sense of self, and self-worth, become intricately bound up with her weight. Weight control becomes a fiercely defended obsession, which may include vomiting and purging.
3 The third stage is reached when the anorexic begins to recognise the addictive nature of her obsession. She realises she is no longer

in control, and begins to look for a way out of the prison she has created for herself.

Although Slade discusses this three-stage model in the context of anorexia, with modification it is a useful framework for thinking about the changes experienced by bulimics. Roughly we are thinking in terms of an early stage before the behaviour has become entrenched, a more advanced stage during which behaviours and attitudes become habitual and the problem denied, and a third stage during which the destructive nature of the behaviour is recognised and the sufferer develops an orientation towards recovery. It is impossible to give a precise time scale to these stages but, as a very rough guide, if stage one has continued for a year or so the condition is likely to run its course through all three stages, which can take up to five years.

Quite specific problems are associated with each stage, hence the sort of help appropriate to each stage will vary. Appropriate help at stage one would involve early identification of the problem and guidance which enables the individual to take steps to avoid the development of the compulsive behaviours characteristic of the second stage. During the second stage there will be considerable disagreement between the sufferer and others (whether these be family and friends or professionals), concerning the nature of her position. During this stage effective service provision may have to be limited to responding to emergencies (in extreme cases this may include hospitalisation). The final stage involves a genuine shift in perception and motivation (seeing there is a problem and wanting to do something about it), and hence offers a major opportunity for providing the sort of assistance which can help the sufferer work towards recovery.

With this three-stage model in mind we can identify three areas in which parents can help:

Recognising early signs
Seeking help
Assisting recovery.

The rest of the chapter will consider each of these areas.

Recognising early signs

Often it is someone other than the anorexic or bulimic who recognises the early signs of an eating disorder. This may be a friend, or parents, or another member of the family. In the early stage the anorexic will not regard her behaviour as a problem. Also many of the associated behaviours will be highly valued by those around her, for example, her determination to lose weight, her devotion to exercise, her self-restraint, her industriousness, etc. There will therefore be a great reluctance to accept that her dieting and weight control are a problem. It is likely to be different for the bulimic as bingeing and vomiting is often accompanied by guilt and is usually kept a secret.

In recent years an increasing amount of attention has been given to the effects of starvation. As we have seen, some authorities in this field have argued that much of the apparently incomprehensible behaviour associated with anorexia and bulimia occurs as a direct result of starvation itself. Although it may be disputed just how significant this factor is, in relation to other factors, starvation is clearly of major importance in accounting for many of the characteristic features of these conditions, especially anorexia. The longer starvation continues the more entrenched the behaviour becomes. Hence the movement from stage one to stage two of Slade's model may occur largely as a result of the increasing effects of starvation, together with the specific forms of reinforcement that contribute to the maintenance of the condition. As we have seen in chapter 3, this process is aptly termed the 'starvation whirlpool' by Roger Slade. It follows from this that the earlier the condition is identified, and help provided, the better.

We have seen that problems related to eating and weight are widespread: 20.6% of women in one recent UK study reported problems in this area. Conflict and struggles related to weight and food are a persistent part of many women's lives. Hence the early stages of anorexia and bulimia will be indistinguishable from behaviour that is apparently very common in our society. However, relatively few women go on to develop the full-blown life-threatening syndromes. So we are looking for signs that may indicate that behaviours which are 'normal' (i.e. common) for young women in our culture are becoming exaggerated and hence characteristic of a serious eating disorder.

Dieting. Of course dieting is very common, and success at dieting is highly valued in our society. Hence initially a woman is likely to be congratulated for her determination to lose weight. But notice if the diet is restricted to a few select foods, such as certain forms of protein (e.g. cheese). Rather than simply reducing or controlling carbohydrate intake anorexics will often seek to eliminate carbohydrate from their diet altogether. They will therefore carefully avoid bread, potatoes, rice, etc. Certain types of food may be met with extreme dislike (e.g. 'I can't stand fish', 'Milk makes me feel sick', 'Bread is revolting'). Despite her own food reduction she may show considerable interest in preparing meals for others and ensuring they eat well. It is not unusual for anorexics to come to exert considerable control over what is cooked and what is eaten in their home. If this tendency is noted it may indicate a growing preoccupation with food intake and body weight which is the hallmark of anorexia and bulimia. It is common for young dieters to experiment with a diet for a few weeks and then drop it. Anorexics don't merely experiment to 'shed a few pounds'. They will stick rigidly to their diet for months on end, and will be very pleased at their obvious success. When they have reached one target weight they will set another. Their dieting becomes relentless. By contrast bulimics often report numerous episodes of dieting which are not as prolonged as the anorexic. The typical patterns in bulimia is for severe dieting to occur in brief episodes followed by increased eating. As a result weight shows considerable fluctuations.

Changes in eating patterns. Such changes may include eating alone, being out, busy, on the phone, or having 'things to do', at meal times; saying she will eat later; tending to avoid social occasions which involve eating, such as visiting relatives. Food may be disposed of secretly: flushed down the toilet, thrown in the dustbin, hidden, or given to the dog. All these may be indications of a growing preoccupation and determination to lose weight that is gradually tending to eclipse all other concerns.

Increased activity. In addition to dieting many anorexics will also exercise intensely in order to lose weight. Also the effects of restricted food intake, plus the sense of control and success as weight falls, can combine to produce a feeling of euphoria. This condition may be comparable to a drug-induced 'high'. As a result it is common to see increased activity and industriousness in the early stages of anorexia. This may involve physical activity or manifest as an increased capacity for homework or revision for exams. Again this is a characteristic that is highly valued in our society and is likely to be strongly reinforced.

Changes in mood and behaviour. The 'high' described in the previous section will often alternate with periods of depression. Being irritable and short-tempered, tending to withdraw to be on her own, and refusing to communicate, will be common features of the 'low' periods. Periods of depression and irritability tend to become more frequent as the condition progresses, often these will be provoked by some perceived lapse in her weight control, or as a result of confrontation with family or friends over her behaviour.

Weight loss. Of course the most obvious external sign of anorexia is weight loss. However it is often very difficult for those in daily contact with the person to recognise the extent of weight loss. It may only be recognised by family or friends who have not seen her for some time. Initially she may be praised or admired for her slender figure. However, as weight loss progresses, family and friends may start to make negative comments. At this stage the anorexic will often go to great lengths to disguise her weight loss, for example through buying larger clothes than she needs and wearing several layers. Early on she may ask you if she looks fat, or says she feels 'too fat' when she is clearly losing weight. Along with weight loss comes an increasing sensitivity to cold, which often leads to disagreements about how high the heating should be at home.

Bingeing. Binge eating often alternates with attempts at dieting, but may occur when the diet is normal. There may be no evidence of weight loss, but evidence of bingeing may be obvious: finding empty food packets in her room; sudden disappearance of food from the kitchen; she may complain she has no money (bingeing can be very expensive); even if the toilet is completely clean evidence of bingeing may be that toilet cleaner goes much quicker that it used to. After meals she may immediately go and spend time in the toilet.

The above features may indicate the development of anorexia or bulimia. But these are certainly insufficient evidence on their own. It must be remembered that difficulties surrounding food and body shape are very common among women in Western societies; but relatively few develop anorexia or bulimia. For parents eager to help there is a real danger of over-reacting. The above guidelines indicate areas where change will occur during the early stages of an eating disorder. But remember very few women will be free of difficulties in these areas. The single most significant piece of evidence that a person has developed a serious eating disorder concerns their attitude to food and weight. If the characteristic 'anorexic attitude' is present there will be several of the features mentioned above. But whereas the above features may be present without a serious threat of anorexia or bulimia the presence of this characteristic attitude should always be treated seriously.

To recap briefly what was said in chapter 2, the 'anorexic attitude' involves an overriding preoccupation with food and weight control, which manifests as a 'relentless pursuit of thinness', and extreme anxiety at the prospect of weight gain. A polarisation occurs between fatness, which becomes equated with what is bad, disgusting, and morally deficient, and thinness which equals good, attractive and pure. An entire life gets built on this equation with thinness pursued relentlessly and compulsively. Weight loss is often accompanied by a sense of triumph and accomplishment, whereas weight gain is responded to with anxiety, depression and despair. This polarisation is the essence of the 'anorexic attitude'. This characteristic attitude will be unmistakable in the advanced stages of anorexia. As starvation progresses this attitude becomes more pronounced and more entrenched; as a result it becomes increasingly hard to modify. Bearing in mind that it is this underlying 'anorexic attitude' which prompts the typical patterns of behaviour of both anorexics and bulimics it will often be apparent in the way a person talks about food and weight, and the intensity of her responses to these issues. Hence this attitude will be apparent even before appreciable weight loss.

Seeking help

The previous section offers some guidelines on early warning signs, but it is by no means easy to identify anorexia or bulimia in the early stages because dieting and weight loss, and bingeing and vomiting, are not unusual behaviours.

In this section we will look at the difficult issue of what to do if you suspect there is a problem. If you are concerned that your daughter may be developing anorexia or bulimia the first thing to do is to **express your concern openly to her**. How to approach the subject with your daughter will depend to a very large extent on the degree to which the problem has developed, and the age of your daughter. What would be an appropriate approach with a 14-year-old in the very early stages of the problem may be completely inappropriate for someone of the same age but whose symptoms have developed to an advanced stage. Further, both of these situations are significantly different, and require correspondingly different approaches, to those involving women in their twenties. Make sure you pick a time when you are calm, and when you know that you and your daughter will have time to talk. The initial approach is best done by focusing on your anxieties. Describe how you feel, and what changes you have actually seen in her behaviour, but do not criticise her, accuse her, blame her, or try to force her to eat. Simply express your feelings of concern and allow her to respond. Try to anticipate what she may say. She may seek to reassure you, or she may get angry, she may accept she has a problem, or she may ignore you; much depends on the nature of your relationship to her, the level of communication and degree of openness in the family. At this stage the goal is to show her your concern and to offer her the opportunity to talk. Do not be deflected from this straightforward goal, avoid slipping into arguments, or pleading with her to change.

Regardless of her response the next stage is to **contact your GP**. It must be borne in mind that the earlier the condition is treated the greater the likelihood of recovery. So if you suspect there is a problem you must seek medical advice as soon as possible. Remember this consultation is for you to talk over your concerns, hence you do not need your daughter's permission. However, do let her know what you are doing so that she gets a clear message that you are concerned. There is often considerable reluctance on the part of parents to acknowledge their daughter may be suffering from anorexia or bulimia. This reluctance is understandable, given the stigma associated with these conditions and given the widespread belief that parents are to blame. Parents must try to overcome these feelings and assess their daughter's behaviour honestly. Further, feelings of shame and anxiety must be overcome in order to go and seek advice from your GP. This is often a very difficult step, but remember the earlier anorexia or bulimia is identified the better the chances of an early recovery. Once developed, say after a year or so, the condition is likely to be firmly established and will then be harder to treat.

When you see your GP. be sure to give as much detail as you can about the behaviours causing you concern. Answer all his or her questions honestly. Your doctor may respond by reassuring you there is nothing to worry about, or he or she may think it advisable to see your daughter personally. Whatever your doctor's response use this opportunity to **ask for information**. Ask if there are any professionals locally who have a special interest in working with anorexics or bulimics. These may be psychiatrists, clinical psychologists, family therapists, social workers, or counsellors. In order to see one of these professionals you may require a written referral from your general practitioner. If it became necessary would he or she provide a referral? Has he or she any idea of the current waiting list for these services? Do any of these offer private sessions? After obtaining information about professional services in your area, ask for information about local self-help groups for anorexics, bulimics and their families.

Now, your GP may well be highly experienced in the area of eating disorders, but you cannot take this for granted. If your GP assures you there is nothing to worry about, and brushes these questions aside, persist. It is advisable for you to obtain this information on what services are available in your area, and how you can avail yourself of them. At this stage you are simply seeking to inform yourself. If your doctor is unhelpful, or you are unsatisfied with his or her response, do not hesitate to go to another doctor. If you have difficulty finding out about local services and self-help groups you can obtain this information through the Eating Disorders Association (their address is provided in appendix 1 at the end of this book).

Over and above finding out about local services, try to find out as much as you can about anorexia and bulimia. Earlier chapters of this book have pointed out that there is considerable controversy about the nature of these conditions, but do not be put off, there is a great deal of useful information available. The books listed in appendix 2 of this book should be all available through public libraries. Self-help groups can provide a wealth of experience and encouragement as well as information about local services (chapter 7 of this book considers self-help groups, and chapter 9 provides an outline of the various types of treatment available). Don't feel you are alone, you will find there are a number of avenues of help open.

Your GP may decide your daughter should be seen for an assessment. He or she may decide to see her personally, or refer her on to a specialist service. If the GP decides to refer to someone else, he or she will send a referral letter outlining the details you have provided, and you will hear from the specialist in due course offering an appointment. Whether it is your GP or a specialist to whom your GP has referred the next task is to **arrange an appointment**. How this is done will of course depend on your daughter's age.

If your daughter is in her early teens or younger, and before extreme weight loss has occurred, it may be sufficient to express your concern about her dieting or weight loss and say you want to go with her to your GP (or a specialist) for a check up. It is important to convey a calm interest in her health, don't criticise her or give the impression that you are frightened. If you receive assurances that she is alright you can reply that you just want to be on the safe side and arrange for her to have a check up. If she is willing, allow her to pick a time. Then make arrangements for the appointment. If you encounter strong resistance you may need to use your authority and insist she attends an appointment. Make arrangements for a time that will be difficult for her to make excuses to miss. Once the appointment has been made **make sure she attends her appointment**. This may not be easy as you may encounter considerable difficulties getting her there. Remain firm and insist that she sees someone, if necessary withdrawing privileges if she seeks to avoid the appointment. This may sound heavy-handed but I want to underline the importance of obtaining professional help early, and of the need for you to demonstrate to her your concern and support.

With older daughters the use of authority will probably not be possible. In these cases your message should nonetheless be clear: you are concerned for her health, and while her health and what she does with her body are her responsibilities, you want her to arrange and attend an appointment, in order for the situation to be properly assessed.

Assisting recovery

There is no magic formula to prevent you saying or doing the wrong thing at times. There is no such think as a perfect parent, hence mistakes are inevitable. Blaming yourself for these mistakes will not help you or your daughter. However it is important to recognise that what you say and do can dramatically affect the course of the illness. This fact can offer considerable grounds for hope: you are not powerless in the face of these conditions.

Parents who have gone through similar experiences, who have often had to learn through painful trial and error, have made a number of recommendations. Many of these suggestions will seem very difficult to apply, and indeed they are, but reports both from those who have suffered anorexia or bulimia, and from their families agree that certain approaches make recovery more likely, while other approaches hinder recovery. The following guidelines indicate the sort of approach which will help create an environment that can assist recovery.

1 Be patient, and don't expect 'miracle cures'. I have stressed the importance of early identification and seeking professional help. For some the duration of the anorexia or bulimia will be relatively brief (less than a year), but for others the condition may last for a number of years. The earlier the condition is identified and help provided the more likely it is that there will be an early recovery, but there can be no guarantee. If the condition has developed to the second stage there will be relatively little that professional helpers can do, at least in the short term. During this second stage especially there is likely to be considerable friction in the family. You may well feel that any professionals involved are not doing enough. During this stage the anorexic or bulimic is likely to refuse treatment or therapy, or to attend appointments with extreme reluctance and resentment. At such times it is natural to blame professionals. The third stage involves genuine change in perception and motivation on the part of the sufferer and offers positive opportunities for recovery. Even so treatment is likely to take a considerable length of time. The hard message is: try to be patient, and do not expect 'miracle cures'.

2 Allow your daughter 'space' for therapy. Assuming your daughter has agreed to see a professional regularly, which may be weekly or fortnightly, the professional will usually want to see your daughter on her own (unless you are attending for family therapy). Whether you accompany her to her appointments will again depend on her age. After the appointment do not try to get your daughter to tell you what she was asked, or what was said, or ask whether she was weighed. If she volunteers information well and good, if she does not that also is fine. Do not try to prise information out of her. Allow her this space and privacy. You may want to consult the professional yourself to ask for advice on how you can best cope with the situation; but resist the temptation to ask for an account of what is happening in the therapy sessions. The professional may contact you to make a specific request or offer suggestions for dealing with the situation. If so it is important to give serious consideration to the recommendations, even if they appear rather drastic (such as withdrawing your daughter from examinations). But here again it is important not to insist on knowing all the details of what has been said during the interviews. I am not saying you do not have a right to be informed about the health of your daughter. Of course you do. But this needs to be balanced against the very great importance of allowing your daughter the opportunity of building a relationship of trust with the person responsible for her therapy. Privacy and confidentiality are absolutely essential in this relationship, and parents can help a great deal when this is respected.

3 Provide love and support. It is very important to show that you love and value your daughter for herself. That is, not because of her achievements, or because she lives up to your expectations, or fulfils your dreams for her, but for herself, as a unique individual. One of the greatest burdens one can carry is to feel you must fulfil the wishes of your parents. Of course you want the best for her but it is essential to demonstrate your love by allowing her to make her own choices and plan her own life. Certainly offer guidance, but don't impose your solutions or your hopes on her. Very often eating disorders develop around the time of exams, or when major life choices have to be made, such as choosing subjects for study in higher education or making career choices. She must learn to make her own way, live her own life, and if necessary make her own mistakes. Never make her feel she has disappointed you. Through all of this difficulty show her your love and support regardless of what she does or doesn't achieve.

4 Listen and communicate. It is important to listen and communicate with your daughter. Talk about anything. Show her you are willing to listen without trying to correct or condemn her. Any talk, no matter how banal, is better than withdrawing and giving her the 'silent treatment'. Make sure you allow communication by listening to her, give her opportunities to express herself honestly, and value her honesty even if you disagree with what she says. Recognise that there are crucial underlying issues beyond food and weight that will need to be dealt with. Allow her to talk about her feelings; and when she does – even if she is expressing hostility – recognise they are her feelings. Never assume you know what she really thinks, feels, or desires. Anorexics and bulimics often have very great difficulty experiencing and expressing their feelings and their needs directly. If you can accept her feelings without panicking, or pretending she doesn't really feel that way, or getting depressed, or blaming her for upsetting you, you will discover feelings are not so dangerous after all. Similarly it is important to allow her to express her thoughts and desires without condemning her, and without trying to change her. This is a very difficult lesson to learn, but a crucial one. It may involve changing the habits of a lifetime.

5 Encourage autonomy. As we have noted anorexia and bulimia appear to be intricately involved with issues of control and autonomy. The process of developing a sense of autonomous identity, and self-worth, require a gradual increase in independence. This raises difficult questions for parents. The one extreme of wanting to do everything for your daughter, to make her decisions, to cling on to her, and the other extreme of pushing her away, blaming her and withdrawing, will both have undesirable consequences. Encourage her to take control of her life without compelling her. Allow yourself to let go without pushing her away. It is understandable that if you see your daughter losing weight, appearing ill and in distress, you will want to take greater control of her life. This understandable response must be resisted. Gently allow her to make her own decisions in as many areas as possible, but do not force her. Your daughter's age will, of course, be a crucial factor determining what would be an appropriate level of independence. In trying to encourage the most appropriate balance between dependence and autonomy, you may find it helpful to discuss this issue with other parents, or someone involved with working with people with eating disorders. A central part of this process is to show respect for her thoughts and feelings, and very importantly to show respect for her privacy. Hence do not open her letters, or read her diaries, or go through her pockets, or cross-examine her friends. Allow her to grow, to become independent, but without pushing her away. Remember that while eating disorders often involve, or express, a struggle for autonomy they also reveal deep-seated anxieties about autonomy. The individual is struggling with deeply conflicting feelings and desires, and they will need continuous encouragement to develop their independence gradually.

6 Set clear boundaries. As important as encouraging autonomy and showing that you love and value your daughter for herself, is the need to set firm boundaries. By this I mean that responsibilities and rights, and what is and is not acceptable behaviour, should be clearly stated. This is true regardless of how old your daughter is, although obviously the age of your daughter will influence the precise nature of the boundaries you set. As long as she lives with you, you have the right to insist on certain standards. When someone becomes ill, for whatever reason, it is accepted that they will be excused certain responsibilities. Going to work or school, doing household chores, taking care of physical needs such as preparing food, looking after clothes, etc., are all areas in which our usual obligations are relaxed when we are ill. Usually family members make allowances for our illness and look after us. However, this temporary relief from normal responsibilities can make being ill quite attractive and this may be a powerful reward, or reinforcement, for being ill. The favourable changes in the family environment brought about because one member is ill, can offer a powerful incentive for that person to remain ill if the gains of illness outweigh the negative aspects of being well.

It is important that you consistently and firmly show that you do not intend to treat your daughter as an invalid, or as 'special' because of her illness. This will mean you do not protect her from the consequences of her behaviour. If your daughter spends all her money on a binge don't increase her allowance, or offer to pay for something she wants. If she makes a mess, perhaps by hiding food somewhere, or by vomiting, insist that she clears it up. You will probably have to struggle with a strong desire to do it for her, but remember that by making allowances and excuses for her you will be rewarding her. Now it may be that she really is too ill to do these things, but if she is you should call your doctor immediately. She may well be upset or angry at your insistence, but obviously this is not the same as being unable to carry out your instructions. If she claims she is too weak, or depressed, or upset to dispose of the bags of food or vomit which she has in her room, point out that she must also be unable to receive phone calls, visit friends, exercise, or do other activities she values. Make her enjoyment of these dependent on her observing basic norms and standards within the family. Remember when you introduce such rules you must give a clear statement of what sanctions will be applied when the rules are broken. Apply sanctions firmly and consistently. If you decide to change rules or sanctions make the changes clear and explain why you are introducing changes. The message she needs to receive is that her illness is not going to be allowed to disrupt the family, or dictate family eating, sleeping or socialising patterns. Her illness must not provide her with an excuse to do whatever she wants. What is and is not acceptable must be clearly stated, and adhered to firmly, even if in the short term you have a fight on your hands.

Don't allow your daughter to manipulate you through threats of harming herself or suicide (but note last paragraph of this chapter). Conflict can become severe, especially if you refuse to allow her illness to dominate the family and dictate what happens at mealtimes. But giving in is always a short-term policy with detrimental effects in the long term. Of course you cannot ignore such threats, but don't allow them to rule your life. Often parents have made dramatic changes in their lives to accommodate their daughter and to avoid 'upsetting her'. This can impose a very severe burden on families and it needs to be firmly resisted. However, this should not be interpreted to mean there ought to be no negotiation. It would certainly be advisable, for example, to negotiate a change in household duties from say shopping or cooking, to something that does not directly involve food. The important thing to remember is that the task may be changed, but she should not be allowed to opt out of all household responsibilities.

These last two points will need to be carefully balanced. I have said you need to respect and encourage your daughter's desire for autonomy, offering support while she struggles with the same issues of identity, self-worth, and personal control. On the other hand you need to set firm boundaries, not treat her as 'special', and try to preserve the normal functioning of the family. The important point is your daughter needs to realise she is special in virtue of her self, not her illness. The precise ways in which you may encourage her growth to independence, and the precise nature of the boundaries you insist on, will of course depend on her age, and will probably vary from family to family. But remember the process of setting clear boundaries will help develop a sense of responsibility, which is a vital part of developing autonomy, and self-identity. The basic principle of encouraging and supporting her growth and maturity, while being firm in order not to reward her illness will need to be thought through in particular cases. The way you apply this principle in specific instances may need to be discussed with your GP, or whoever is seeing your daughter for therapy. There is no doubt that the required blend of concern and love, coupled with firmness, is a difficult balance to achieve. But it is also clear that one without the other will usually make the situation worse.

To conclude this point a word of warning: do not make rules or attempt to apply sanctions over food. Remember this section is about helping your daughter to experience a sense of responsibility for her actions. This involves refusing to protect her from the consequences of her behaviour. It is also about minimising the impact of anorexia or bulimia on family functioning.

But note that it is absolutely essential that you do not attempt to make rules or apply sanctions specifically to her eating behaviour.

7 Don't make an issue out of food or weight. I have emphasised the importance of being firm with respect to what is acceptable behaviour, not allowing her illness to function as an excuse. But the area in which you must show allowances and be flexible is the issue of food itself. It will not help if you try to force her to eat or insist on weighing her. If she wants to eat alone let her. Do not make an issue out of it. Let her make her own decisions about food. The reason why you should not try to 'lay down the law' with respect to food intake is that with anorexics and bulimics food and weight become the focus of very powerful feelings of fear and guilt. If you try to exert your authority and force her to eat a particular amount, food will become a family battleground which will only serve to exacerbate the problem. Don't try to scare her into eating by telling her stories of people who have died from anorexia. I have known instances where such shock tactics appear to have had the effect of preventing the development of anorexia, but this occurred early in the first stage of the condition, and I know of many more where the 'shock tactics' have had precisely the opposite effect. Also it appears that many anorexics learn to use vomiting as a way of getting rid of unwanted food after having been bullied into eating food they did not want.

To summarise this point: concerning the specific issues of food intake, and weight, it is advisable to be flexible and tolerant. Avoid confrontations on these issues. Recognise your daughter is not just being awkward, she is terrified of gaining weight. However, as noted in point 6, do put firm limits on the extent to which her illness is allowed to encroach on to the everyday functioning of the family. She may be terrified of eating, but she is not terrified of doing her share of chores, or clearing up mess she has made. On these other areas be firm: don't reward her illness by letting her opt out of family responsibilities.

8 Don't punish her for being ill. In setting clear boundaries it is important to recognise you are not attempting to punish her for her illness. You are not making her do things she wouldn't do if she were well. Setting boundaries should not be used as a means of punishing her. Remember anorexia and bulimia are serious disorders which involve considerable emotional distress for the sufferers. It will not help if you attempt to impose punishments on her for refusing to eat, or for vomiting. Do not blame her, or accuse her of destroying the family or ruining your life. Emotional blackmail will not work; she undoubtedly has enough anxiety and guilt already.

9 Learn how to deal with conflict. Disagreement and conflict within the family are inevitable, but families deal with conflict very differently. Bear in mind that the expression of anger is not necessarily a bad thing, provided you observe certain constraints. While you may justifiably be angry about your daughter's actions, never allow yourself to criticise her. Assume she had vomited over the table during a meal. You may justifiably express your anger about this action, and make her clear it up, but do not accuse her of being selfish, or wilful, or impossible. You may criticise what she has done, but you should not criticise her as a person. 'You have made a mess and spoilt the meal for everyone else, now clear it up,' is a very different form of criticism to, 'You're the most selfish person I know, what have we done to deserve a daughter like you?'

Remember she may appear to be a tyrant at times, exerting tremendous power over the family in various ways, but beneath this her self-esteem, even her sense of self-identity, will be very fragile. She is probably racked with guilt, and self-loathing. So try to distinguish between her actions, which you may justifiably criticise, and herself which you should never criticise.

It is equally important to resist the temptation to try to control her behaviour through emotional blackmail. Don't say: 'After all we've done for you', 'You're not the girl you used to be', 'We were such a happy family', 'Look what you're doing to us, you're making your father ill', 'What have we done to deserve this?', 'You're not my daughter'. These sorts of remarks will certainly make her feel worse and are very unlikely to improve the situation.

10 Don't encourage her 'anorexic attitude'. As we have seen the driving force behind anorexia and bulimia is a particular attitude towards body weight in which thinness comes to have a significance intricately related to the individual's sense of self. As starvation progresses this attitude becomes more exaggerated and more entrenched. The really difficult task in the process of recovery is not putting on weight, or even stopping bingeing, it is rather the abandoning of the anorexic attitude. This is the heart of the problem. Part of the reason this step is so difficult is because the roots of the 'anorexic attitude', or 'anorexic thinking', is an exaggeration of views widely held in our culture. In talking with anorexics I have often been struck by the fact that their position can follow with impeccable logic from premises widely accepted in our society. Praising thinness, buying diet books, dieting yourself, or in any way contributing to the view that fat equals bad, and thin equals good, will reinforce her attitude. Also recognise that as anorexia develops perceptual distortions can become pronounced, it is important not to collude with her by agreeing with her perceptions. Try to express your disagreement calmly, not expecting to change her mind, but simply to convey that you do not see things as she does. Included in this would be a willingness to acknowledge your own mistakes. Anorexics and bulimics are often perfectionists with little tolerance of shortcomings. Show her you do not expect perfection of yourself, or of her. It is also important not to collude with her by pretending she isn't thin, or denying she is bingeing or vomiting. Don't put a veil of silence over these things.

11 A consistent approach. It is important that both parents discuss and agree on how to respond to their daughter's illness. Alliances, with one parent taking their daughter's side against the other, are often very destructive. It is common for this to occur and for one parent to withdraw from the situation. Make sure there is regular communication so you can give your daughter consistent messages about your concern and love for her, and what aspects of her behaviour you will and will not accept. This is often extremely difficult to do. It is not unusual for one parent, very often the father, to withdraw and expect their spouse to cope with the situation. This will create divisions within the family which is likely to impede recovery. It is essential that both parents be involved.

12 Look after yourself and your marriage. Your daughter's struggle with anorexia or bulimia will be your struggle also. It may turn out to be an arduous journey spanning several years.

Hence, you *must* look after yourself and your marriage. You will not be able to help your daughter if your marriage is undermined or one or both of you are failing to cope at work or with domestic responsibilities. In addition to finding out what help is available for your daughter, it is essential that you are aware of what help is available for you. You will need advice and support. Lots of it. Chapter 7 of this book is devoted to self-help and contains information on self-help groups; these groups offer an invaluable source of help to both sufferers and their families. But, in addition, if the stress of coping with your anorexic or bulimic daughter becomes too great then contact your GP and ask for a referral to a professional who can help you with stress management. Just as there is no reason why you should feel ashamed that your daughter has anorexia or bulimia you should not be ashamed of asking for help if the stress becomes too great.

Emergency situations

In conclusion, a word about emergency situations. Both anorexia and bulimia can lead to physical complications which can be fatal. Death from starvation can sometimes result from anorexia. Also both anorexics and bulimics can become so distressed that there is a serious risk of suicide. If your daughter talks about killing herself you must take this seriously. Although the threat of suicide may be employed as a way of controlling other people you must obtain a professional opinion and not try to assess the seriousness of the situation on your own. If your daughter says she wants to kill herself notify your GP and her therapist immediately. Also if you have reason to doubt whether her therapist is monitoring her physical condition properly make enquiries and express your reasons for concern clearly. If your daughter faints or is so weak she is unable to walk you must call the emergency services immediately, even if she insists she is all right, or gets angry. Although it is a minority of anorexics and bulimics whose difficulties reach the stage where life is seriously threatened, it is important to be aware of the possibility, and to make sure you do not try to deal with these situations on your own.

6 How can relatives, partners and friends help?

Many anorexics and bulimics are young women, often in their teens, living with their parents. In the last chapter we considered the problems facing parents who are trying to respond to the stresses and demands of this situation. We also noted the difficulties facing parents with an anorexic or bulimic daughter who no longer lives with them. But of course it is not just parents who will want to offer help. Other members of the family are often closely involved: brothers, sisters, aunts, uncles, etc. Often there will be friends keen to offer their help. Also there are situations where parents are not closely involved, perhaps where the anorexic or bulimic lives with relatives, or with a friend, or spouse, or a sexual partner, or alone. There may be situations where the parents have deliberately withdrawn, or their daughter may have chosen to distance herself from them. The situations in which anorexics and bulimics find themselves are varied, and the people closely involved may range from grandparents to friends.

Our personal relationships can bring great pleasure, satisfaction and fulfilment, or they can be a source of pain, fear and despair. Anorexics and bulimics often describe serious difficulties in their relationships with others. Along with a feeling that personal contacts are unrewarding and unsatisfactory, there is often a tendency to withdraw and isolate themselves. This tendency is greatly amplified as anorexia or bulimia becomes more severe. Part of the reason for this progressive withdrawal from other people is the impact of starvation on psychological functioning. As we have seen in chapter 3, starvation exaggerates distortions in thinking and reduces flexibility of thought. When the characteristic 'anorexic attitude' becomes pronounced and entrenched, communication becomes very difficult. As a result not only does the anorexic or bulimic tend to withdraw, but others may also find it very difficult to be with them and hence may withdraw themselves.

We have noted that anorexia and bulimia often involve

problems associated with establishing a clear sense of self, and of developing a capacity for autonomous action. Now, one of the most important ways of establishing a sense of identity is through relationships with others. Through our relationships we develop not just a sense of who we are, but also an impression of our worth, or value. Our sense of self-identity, and our self-esteem, are crucially related to the quality of our personal relationships. Also our capacity to act independently, or autonomously, develops in the context of relationships. Difficulties in personal relationships can actually facilitate the development of a sense of self if those difficulties are resolved or overcome. However withdrawal from others will preclude such development. Anorexics and bulimics are in great need of supportive relationships. So, although it may sound trite, the most valuable form of help that you can offer an anorexic or bulimic is genuine friendship.

In chapter 5 it was noted that parents may help their anorexic or bulimic daughters in three general areas: recognising early signs, seeking help, and assisting recovery. Many of the principles and suggestions given in chapter 5 will also apply to those whose relationship to the sufferer is not that of parents. However, there are important differences. For example, it was noted in chapter 5 that parents with a young daughter may appropriately use their authority to ensure she attends an appointment with a GP or specialist. In this respect parents with a young daughter are in a unique position. With older daughters using such authority becomes progressively harder, and of course progressively more inappropriate. The situation is very different if it is your friend, your sister, your spouse, your sexual partner, or a daughter who now lives independently from you, whom you suspect is becoming anorexic or bulimic. This chapter will outline guidelines for dealing with these situations. The material in this chapter should be read along with chapter 5, as many of the points in that chapter are relevant to these situations also. Once again I would like to repeat what was said at the beginning of chapter 5. There are no hard and fast rules that will guarantee you say or do exactly what is needed at the right time. Individuals, situations, and relationships vary so much that the best that can be done is to provide guidelines that will need to be thought through carefully when applied to specific cases. In particular the changes that are likely to occur in the course of anorexia or bulimia must be taken into account when you apply these suggestions. The first section of chapter 5 outlines these changes using Peter Slade's three-stage model. The information below should be read bearing in mind the different responses likely at different stages of the condition.

1 Express your concern. Information on identifying early signs has been given in chapter 5. Often friends or partners are able to notice changes in weight, eating habits, dieting, mood and behaviour, etc., very early on. As was suggested with parents the first step is to express your concern to the person directly. Regardless of whether you are a friend, a brother or sister, a spouse or partner, it is important to state your concerns clearly. In doing this keep three aims clearly in mind: first, describe the behaviours that cause you concern, remember stick to what you have seen or heard her say, do not make guesses; second, express how you feel about the situation; third, give her the opportunity to express herself.

Once again I must emphasise it will not help if you approach her when you are angry or upset. Remain calm. Do not try to blame her, or blackmail her, or accuse her. Do not try to persuade her to eat, or to tell you her weight, or to let you weigh her, or to tell you how often she is bingeing and vomiting. Your objective is to voice your concerns without driving her away.

2 Encourage her to see a therapist. Once the issue has been brought out into the open she may accept she has a problem and agree to seek help. However, she may try to convince you that you are over-reacting, she may become angry, or she may get upset. You are now in the very difficult position of having to decide how serious the problem is. You may be over-reacting; or you may not. I strongly recommend you seek professional advice. Be very clear on what you have seen that causes you concern and talk it over with someone who knows about eating disorders. If it is your partner you are concerned about, approach your GP. If it is a fellow student, talk to the university doctor or counsellor. If it is a school friend, talk to a teacher. The professional you speak to may feel there is nothing to worry about, or they may want to see her themselves. What happens next will vary, depending on the situation and the professional

D

you consult. They may choose to visit her, or you may be asked if you could encourage her to contact them.

Remember: the sooner therapy is provided the better the chances of an early recovery. Hence, it is important to encourage her to see her doctor, or therapist, or a counsellor. But she may refuse. Unless the problem has reached a stage where her physical health is endangered, or unless there is a risk of suicide, you will not be able to override her wishes and make sure she is seen by her doctor against her will. You must respect her wishes and it will not help to keep on about it or try to force her into therapy.

Friends often experience great conflict when they must decide whether to inform parents, school or university authorities of their friend's eating problem. Loyalty to a friend and concern for her wellbeing appear to conflict. However, it must be remembered that anorexia and bulimia are serious problems, and receiving help is essential. She may be angry with you initially but if she receives help soon as a result of your action you may be saving her a lot of suffering, and perhaps even saving her life.

3 Don't try to control her eating. Whether she is your wife, lover, sister or friend, and whether she is in therapy or not, her weight and her eating are her business. Do not try to control her eating or her weight. You will not be able to force her to eat, or stop her bingeing and vomiting. But you can certainly make her a lot worse through trying to control her. It is even unwise to make suggestions about what she should or should not eat, or what weight she should or should not be. Also be careful that you do not try to control her eating indirectly by commenting on her appearance. She will need to come to terms with her difficulties herself, and you can be of great help if you allow her to make her own choices about what she eats and how she controls her weight. She will be helped by your love and friendship not by your attempts to control her eating.

4 Let her be responsible for her behaviour. As with parents there is a risk that partners, wanting to protect their spouse or lover, will encourage them to relinquish responsibilities. But it is very important that this is resisted. You may choose to renegotiate household chores or responsibilities in the relationship, taking into account her problems with food, but the renegotiation should be fair with responsibilities balanced on both sides. Hence, you may decide that you should take responsibility for household food money and food purchases, but if this was originally your partner's responsibility it will be fair for her to take over some of your chores. You may feel very sorry for her, but it will not help if you encourage her to opt out of her responsibilities. Do not treat your partner as an invalid, or a helpless child.

Another aspect of allowing an anorexic or bulimic person to be responsible for their behaviour, concerns taking steps to reduce the impact her behaviour has on others. Although you will not be able to make her eat or stop her bingeing or vomiting, you can certainly act to reduce the disruption her behaviour has on you and others in the household. For example you may share a flat with a friend you suspect is bulimic. You may be very annoyed with the mess she leaves in the bathroom, or the amount of food that is disappearing from the kitchen. In such situations it is important to express your dissatisfaction to your friend and discuss arrangements to deal with the problem; such as buying food separately. Do not ignore such problems, and resist the temptation to do things for her, such as clearing up mess she has made. Similarly it is unwise to alter your eating habits to accommodate her problem. If you decide not to buy certain foods that you like because you know they will tempt your flatmate or spouse to binge, you will not be helping her. The general principle is that while you should not try to control her eating behaviour, you can and should try to reduce its impact on you. This will have two important effects. First, you will find you will be able to cope much better with the stress of living with someone who has anorexia or bulimia when you are able to control the level of disruption occurring in your household. Second, you will be demonstrating that you believe she can behave responsibly, and indeed, expect her to do so.

5 Don't blame her, or her mother. It is common to find people blaming the anorexic or bulimic person ('She's just being awkward', 'She's just too lazy to try'), or blaming her mother ('If you met her mother you would know why she is like that'). Apart from being unreasonable such attitudes are extremely unhelpful. Instead of looking for someone to blame, it is far more productive to focus on developing the sort of relationship that will contribute to her recovery.

6 Focus on your relationship with her, not her eating. I have stressed the importance of allowing the person with anorexia or bulimia to make their own choices about food and weight control. As you do this you will naturally withdraw attention from her weight and what she is eating. Obviously you will be concerned not to give the impression that you no longer care. While it is wise to let her decide what she will eat, and what weight she wants to be, it is important for you to try to cultivate your relationship with her. The goal is for you to relate to her, not her eating habits. It is common for an eating disorder to become the central feature of a relationship. All interactions become somehow undermined by the 'problem with food and weight'. But try to put the fact that she is anorexic or bulimic to one side, and see her as a person again. Show that you value the relationship and won't allow her difficulties with food to destroy it. This will mean listening to her and communicating with her regularly. It will mean spending time together. There will be some activities that may present difficulties such as shopping together or going out for a meal. In these cases do not assume you know how she will react: ask her. She may say she would rather not eat out, if so that's fine. There are many other things you can do together. Work to improve your relationship and enjoy your time together. Let her work through her eating problems, you cannot do it for her.

7 Don't try to be her therapist. When you do not pressure her to eat, or focus on her problem, you may find she wants to talk to you about her difficulties, or about her therapy. This can be of great help to her as long as you don't try to undermine her therapy, or try to tell her how to solve her problems. If she wants to talk listen carefully, and try to support and encourage her. It will be helpful if you can inform yourself about anorexia and bulimia through reading and perhaps through attending a self-help group. But remember: what she does about her eating and her weight is her responsibility; and you are not her therapist. Be what you are: her friend, her sister, her husband, or her lover.

8 Make sure you are not using her problem as a diversion. Sometimes an eating disorder can come to be the major focus of attention in a relationship. If your partner is anorexic and you find it impossible to follow the guidelines given above, which

suggest shifting attention from her eating to improving your relationship, then it may be the case that the problem with eating is being used as a diversion. Perhaps there are other aspects of your relationship that are in serious need of attention, but are difficult for you and your partner to address. Perhaps there is a sexual problem, or problem with children, or some other major area of conflict. In these cases the eating problem may be maintained because it is less threatening than facing other issues. Although it appears that it is the person with anorexia or bulimia that has 'the problem', sometimes her partner may use her difficulties with food as a way of avoiding his own problems – which may be to do with areas of his life that his anorexic or bulimic partner is scarcely aware of. These situations can be extremely complex, hence if you find it impossible to disentangle yourself from your partner's eating it would be advisable to seek professional help.

9 Be prepared for change. As someone recovers from anorexia or bulimia they will make changes in areas of their life other than food and weight. You may find your friend or partner starts to express her thoughts, feelings and preferences in a more assertive way. You may find she moves towards greater independence and begins to exert a greater level of control over her life. Such changes are an essential part of the recovery process and, while you may find such changes challenging, it is important to recognise that they indicate she is beginning to come to terms with the conflicts and problems that underlie the eating disorder, and hence such changes will need to be encouraged. If you find it difficult to accept these changes, or feel they undermine your relationship, once again it is advisable to bring your anxieties out into the open and talk to your friend or partner.

10 Look after yourself. As has been pointed out with respect to parents, although you may feel alone and unsupported, there are a number of sources of help available. It is essential for you to obtain support, guidance and encouragement. This may be found through talking to your GP, a therapist or a counsellor. But another avenue of support that may be available locally is a self-help group. Self-help groups are available not just for sufferers from anorexia and bulimia, but for their relatives, friends and partners. How to find out where the groups meet, what they do, and how they can benefit attenders, are discussed in the next chapter.

7 Self-help

This chapter will focus on the area of self-help, not just for the anorexic and bulimic but also for their families and friends. We will consider self-help groups first and then look at self-help strategies. But before we do this there are two essential preliminary points to be emphasised.

Personal responsibility

Throughout this book I have emphasised the point that anorexia and bulimia are serious problems that require professional help, whether from a GP, psychiatrist, clinical psychologist, psychotherapist, or counsellor. Professional help may also be needed by parents, partners, or others closely involved with a sufferer. However, it is clearly not the case that professionals can 'make people better'. The capacity and power for recovery lies within the individual sufferer, and nowhere else. If someone enters therapy in the belief that the therapist will 'sort everything out', they are bound to be disappointed. A therapist can provide guidance, encouragement and support, and help mobilise a person's inner resources and capacity for change. This form of help can make a substantial difference but only if it meets with a positive response. The therapist is responsible for providing a service, or providing informed help, but the responsibility and power for change remains with the client. Dawn, a recovered anorexic, told me: 'For years people just seemed to me to be interfering and incompetent. No-one seemed to understand me, but I really didn't mind. I always knew, at the back of my mind, that nothing would change until I wanted it to.'

Personal responsibility for change may be readily accepted, but what is often harder to accept is personal responsibility for one's suffering. This involves accepting responsibility not only for our actions but also for our feelings, distress, and symptoms. Of course, it is certainly possible to argue persuasively that the position we find ourselves in has occurred, at least in part, through processes over which we have no control. We have seen socio-cultural factors appear to play a part in the aetiology of eating problems. However, it is important to recognise that engagement in therapy and recovery are very difficult for any-one who persists in seeing themselves as passive victims of situations or processes over which they have no control. Accept-ing responsibility for our difficulties does not mean blaming ourselves or saying we are at fault. Rather it means acknow-ledging that our distress, our problems, our symptoms, are ours, and that ultimately we are the only ones who can over-come them. The philosophy of self-help involves recognising that while others can help, they cannot 'make us well'. 'Self-help' involves availing oneself of all possible assistance, recog-nising and valuing other people's knowledge and experience, but at the same time accepting the often unpalatable fact that we alone are ultimately responsible for ourselves.

'Underlying issues'

As we have seen in chapters 1 to 4, there are substantial differences of opinion regarding the nature, definition and causes of anorexia and bulimia. However, there is wide agree-ment that preoccupations with food and weight loss, and binge-eating and purging, are expressions, or symptoms, of 'underly-ing' problems which must be addressed if genuine recovery is to occur. Accounts of the nature of these underlying problems vary, but difficulties usually centre on issues such as: the need to establish a sense of self-identity; problems with low self-esteem; desires for autonomy, independence, personal effective-ness and control over one's life, which may conflict with desires for nurturance, dependence, security and closeness; dealing with the demands and expectations of others, and personal perfectionism; coping with stress and difficult feelings.

Throughout this book, and indeed throughout the literature on anorexia and bulimia these and related issues occur time and time again. Many features of 'self-help' facilitate change in these areas and serve to address these issues rather than specifically food and weight. In many self-help groups there is an explicit commitment to the view that difficulties with body weight and food intake will resolve if progress can be made in these areas of 'underlying', or 'existential' concern.

Self-help groups

In the last 20 years there has been a rapid growth in the number of self-help groups covering a very wide range of issues and problems. In Britain you can find self-help groups for alcoholics and for their children and spouses; for victims of sexual abuse, and for the perpetrators; for relatives of people suffering incapacitating conditions such as dementia, and schizophrenia; for sufferers from cancer, and their relatives; for the bereaved; for carers of people with learning difficulties; for gamblers, and many more.

Self-help groups have been defined as: 'groups of people who feel they have a common problem and have joined together to do something about it.' So self-help groups are comprised of people who are united by virtue of sharing a common problem. People will be at different stages, some may well have recovered completely, but group members have the opportunity to share their experiences and thereby help one another. Some of these function independently but most are associated with larger organisations. In Britain at present the largest network of self-help groups for anorexics and bulimics and their families is affiliated to the Eating Disorders Association. This organisation was founded in 1989 when Anorexic Aid and The Anorexic Family Aid National Information Centre were merged. The Eating Disorders Association co-ordinates a network of over 30 self-help groups in Britain. (The association provides a range of services including telephone help-lines and information on local professional and voluntary services. The address of the Eating Disorder Association, and the numbers of their help-lines are given in appendix 1 at the end of this book.) Broadly speaking self-help groups provide two forms of help: advice and support. They do not provide therapy, or offer a substitute for therapy.

What actually happens at a self-help group? As there are many groups operating in Britain there is considerable variation in the way meetings are organised. Some groups may prefer a fairly open format. That is, apart from a very brief introduction from one member covering any business the group may need to attend to (such as forthcoming events of interest to the group, any financial issues, etc.), the groups will be open for members to raise whatever issues they want. There may be requests for information or advice, or expressions of difficulties, or any other topic of concern to individual members. There will usually be a group leader, or facilitator. This may be the person who originally established the group, but more often this role will rotate, as members feel more able and willing to be involved.

Even with groups associated with the Eating Disorders Association there will be variations in format, depending on the needs and decisions of each group. However, Pat Hartley, a psychologist working in Manchester and founder of Anorexic Aid, has suggested the following outline:

1 Self-introduction by facilitators and members, each perhaps declaring the nature of her involvement.
2 Any group business or announcement of future activities.
3 A clear statement of group goals and 'rules', especially if new members are present.
4 A short presentation by member or invited speaker chosen from topics such as:
   (a) Effective goals and coping strategies.
   (b) Perfectionism.
   (c) Sex-role stereotyping.
   (d) Guilt.
   (e) Pleasurable alternatives to dieting and bingeing.
   (f) Family dynamics.
   (g) Medical complications of starving, bingeing and purging.
   (h) Anger and rage. Forms of expression.
   (i) Personal accounts by recovered anorexics or bulimics.
5 A discussion of the presentation, perhaps in subgroups.
6 A feedback session involving the full group.
7 Conclusion – involving opportunity for members to exchange telephone numbers and addresses or to arrange individual meetings; discussion of other issues relevant to members. A selection of leaflets, booklists or books for loan may be available for members before and after the main part of the meeting.

Frequency and duration of meetings also varies, but usually they will be bi-weekly or weekly, lasting from one hour, to an hour and a half.

Benefits of self-help groups

Some of the positive benefits claimed for self-help groups are set out below.

Reduction of isolation. Anorexics and bulimics usually come to feel extremely isolated. This will occur for many reasons. The disturbances in thinking, outlined in chapter 3, gradually become more entrenched as anorexia or bulimia develops. In particular the dramatic polarisation of thinking around the central obsession with body weight makes communication very difficult, both for the sufferer and for those who try to communicate with her. This difficulty in communication often leads to reduced social contacts and withdrawal.

Often the isolation of the anorexic is of someone who feels disconnected from others by virtue of her uniqueness. Anorexics are often described as 'proud and aloof'. Many experience a sense of superiority, frequently of moral superiority, when they are successfully losing weight. Beneath this superior attitude there are usually profound feelings of worthlessness, which rapidly manifest when she experiences problems with weight control. But whether she is feeling superior, or worthless, there will be considerable problems interacting with others.

Bulimia often provokes severe feelings of shame, guilt and self-disgust, and is usually kept secret from others. This sense of being fundamentally unacceptable, even 'disgusting' (a term often used by bulimics themselves to describe their behaviour), is often accompanied by depression which can be very serious – risk of suicide is not uncommon. These feelings will all tend to make someone suffering from bulimia withdraw from social contacts.

But it is certainly not just the sufferers from anorexia and bulimia who experience this isolation: family members, parents and partners in particular, often share a sense of being alone, of having to struggle with apparently intractable problems without guidance or support. It is common for families to look inward and reduce their social contacts as they become dominated by the anxieties and problems of their daughter's condition.

Self-help groups provide an opportunity to break out of this isolation and meet others with very similar difficulties. For both sufferers and their families recognising that others have been in similar situations and have managed, not merely to survive the ordeal, but have actually learnt and grown through it, can be an enormously powerful and encouraging experience.

Information. Self-help groups often provide a rich source of information, not just in terms of understanding anorexia and bulimia, but also concerning local services. Self-help groups often include members with experience of various local agencies, and have had contacts with various therapists and counsellors. What professional help is available; who offers what sort of therapy; and perhaps particular recommendations of who can help and who should be avoided, can often be provided by people with first-hand experience. Although there are now many books on anorexia and bulimia which are readily available, specific information on local services is not so easily obtained, hence this aspect of self-help groups is extremely valuable.

Practical suggestions. As well as information people often want advice. That is, practical suggestions for dealing with specific problems. Written material can help but as each situation is unique, it may be difficult to see how to apply suggestions to your own situation. Self-help groups often contain a wealth of understanding and experience that cannot be found in books. Being able to discuss issues with people who have been in similar, though of course not identical, situations can provide new perspectives and options that may be of great help. Often practical suggestions will centre on 'coping strategies', and include areas such as those noted in the meeting outline suggested by Pat Hartley, given above. Techniques of problem-solving, coping with feelings, understanding family interactions, etc., are various ways of increasing coping ability and reducing stress and as such they can play an important part in the process of recovery.

Credible role models. In terms of Peter Slade's three-stage model outlined in chapter 5, self-help groups may be of considerable value to someone in the early stages of an eating disorder because they offer an opportunity to see and hear from those who have experienced the advanced stages of these conditions.

Advice or information offered to someone in the early stages of anorexia or bulimia may often go unheeded if it comes from parents or a GP. The person feels 'got at', and may feel an increasing sense of distance and misunderstanding between herself and such authority figures. By contrast receiving information, advice or support from a contemporary, who may well express similar anxieties and conflicts, is often accepted as 'authoritative' in a way that communications from parents or professionals are not. Seeing others in more advanced stages of emaciation, and identifying her own condition in what is said, can be a powerful stimulus to act in such a way as to prevent the condition developing any further.

In the advanced stage of anorexia or bulimia, in which the behaviour has become entrenched but is now perceived as a problem for which the sufferer needs help, self-help groups can offer an invaluable source of advice and support. The addictive nature of advanced anorexia and bulimia make it very difficult to alter the established patterns of behaviour. Hearing how others have worked to free themselves; how others deal with setbacks and cope with emergencies; and hearing about the process of recovery, etc., can be a powerful source of encouragement, and reinforce efforts to change.

Acceptance and support. As group participants are united by virtue of having experienced similar struggles, self-help groups provide a context in which problems and setbacks are received non-judgementally. Hence participants are not merely encouraged and reinforced for accomplishments and successes, they also receive valuable emotional support when in the midst of difficulties. This is a very important feature of self-help groups because anorexics, bulimics, and their families, are often extremely self-critical and frequently suffer intense feelings of guilt. Receiving acceptance and understanding from others who have experienced similar feelings can encourage the self-acceptance, and self-tolerance, that is so essential for recovery.

Empowerment. One of the major issues believed to underlie anorexia and bulimia is the challenge of autonomy; that is, developing a capacity for free and independent action. When movement towards autonomy is opposed by feelings of inadequacy, anxiety, fear or guilt, conflict results. This conflict can produce what Hilde Bruch called 'the paralysing sense of ineffectiveness', which often characterises anorexia and bulimia. Encouraging and supporting autonomy is a crucial part of the recovery process. The essential first step in this process is the recognition and acceptance of personal responsibility. Without this acceptance of responsibility genuine autonomous action is impossible. Self-help groups can greatly facilitate autonomy by encouraging members to accept responsibility for change, and emphasising the fact that change is possible.

Accepting personal responsibility is the first step in acting autonomously. It is also the first step to 'empowerment'. What I mean by that term is the feeling, or conviction, that one's behaviour, thoughts, feelings, life situation, relationships, and even symptoms, are not imposed upon one as unalterable facts. Many people find the practical guidance and encouragement provided through a self-help group helps increase their sense of mastery over their lives. Many anorexics then begin to experience a sense of effectiveness that is not based purely on their ability to lose weight. This is an absolutely crucial shift. If she can feel effective, or powerful in areas other than that of food and weight control, her psychological survival, or sense of self, will no longer be exclusively rooted in her body shape. She may then be able to relax control of her eating and weight. Often the professional approach to anorexia and bulimia involves exerting control over the sufferer 'for her own good'. In the case of anorexia the more severe the weight loss, the more intrusive the treatment. Regardless of the motives of the professional this exercise of power necessarily entails reducing the control and autonomy of the sufferer. I do not want to imply that such intrusions are never justified; it can certainly be argued that someone in the grip of the advanced stages of anorexia or bulimia is far from being in control. But there is an inherent contradiction in attempting to help someone locked in a personal struggle which involves issues of control by reducing their sense of control still further. Self-help does offer a considerable advantage by putting responsibility and control into the hands of sufferers.

Role reversal. The group provides a context in which the experience of anorexia and bulimia, and the issues surrounding these conditions, are taken seriously. The individual's struggle is not only understood, it is also valued. Members can develop a sense of self-worth and increase self-esteem as they develop their understanding of the role food and weight plays in their lives, and as they begin to tackle the intricate process of recovery. Of major importance is the principle of 'helper therapy'. That is, as the member gains confidence and begins to value what she has learnt in the course of her struggle she will communicate with, and learn to support, others. This process will tend to consolidate her own gains. In helping others she helps herself. Many anorexics and bulimics have described profound changes occurring in their lives when they move from being a passive receiver of advice, support or help, to being an active provider. This feature of self-help groups is another means by which the individual can experience herself as effective, that is, 'role reversal' is another move towards empowerment.

Reservations about self-help groups

For the reasons given in this chapter self-help groups can play an important part in recovery. However, it is important to note there have been criticisms, and reservations, expressed about self-help groups. I will outline some of the more important ones.

Symptom reinforcement. Some concern has been expressed that self-help groups may reinforce weight loss by encouraging competition among anorexics as to who can be the thinnest. As far as one can judge from information provided by members of self-help groups, this rarely occurs. We have noted in chapter 2 the tendency for anorexics to perceive their body as being larger than it is. However, this misperception does not occur in respect to other people. Hence the group member may be shocked by the degree of emaciation of other members, and even more shocked when they hear they are as thin or thinner. The group medium therefore may facilitate correction of perceptual distortions and help clarify the seriousness of their problem. It has also been suggested that members can learn new ways of losing weight, or concealing their behaviours, or manipulating therapists, through what they hear in the groups. There is certainly a possibility of this happening, especially for those in the first two stages of anorexia or bulimia. But this risk needs to be balanced against the powerful influence towards recovery that can be present in a self-help group.

Lack of evaluation. There has been very little evaluation of self-help groups. Research so far has largely focused on finding out what features of the self-help group members feel have been helpful. This type of research may be useful but does not offer any comparative information. However, anecdotal evidence suggests self-help groups have played a key role in the process of recovery.

Variation between groups. As we have seen, part of the self-help philosophy involves giving members the responsibility for setting the format of the meetings. This inevitably results in variation between groups. Given this flexibility there is scope for individual groups to develop idiosyncratic characteristics. Some of which may not be helpful to members. Hence competition and rivalry can develop, as can group 'norms' which can be moralistic and off-putting to new members. Given the philosophy of self-help groups it would be inappropriate to impose a rigid structure on all groups, hence local variations are inevitable. It should be borne in mind therefore that if you attend a group which does not meet your needs, or is not to your liking for some reason, this does not mean that self-help groups are not for you. Remember the groups will vary. Some will have 10 to 20 regular and active attenders, other groups will be comparatively small and inactive. Find out what groups are in your area and try them.

Avoidance of therapy. Another problem which can arise is that members may regard the group as an alternative to therapy, and hence have high expectations of what the group can offer. Although in this chapter I have given a largely positive account of self-help groups it is important to see their role as complementing individual therapy rather than as an alternative. In some cases an anorexic or bulimic may attend a group because little is demanded of her and she therefore sees it as an easy option and a way of avoiding therapy. One anorexic told me she attended a self-help group for a year: 'just to keep mum and dad off my back'.

Group authority. Some people may experience groups as authoritarian and oppressive. There is no doubt that groups can exert great power over group members. However, once again we need to balance the fact that some people will experience the authority of the group in a negative way with the evidence that suggests that others experience the groups authority in a very positive and supportive way.

Over-dependence. Some may feel groups encourage dependency and as such oppose genuine movements towards autonomy. This is certainly a pitfall that needs to be guarded against, but evidence does indicate that most group members go through a period of dependency on the group initially, then as recovery progresses there is a gradual increase in independence and a reduction in reliance on the group.

Many recovered anorexics and bulimics have commented that their experience of therapy or treatment often focused unduly on food and weight and not enough on such underlying issues as self-identity, control, autonomy, family and sexual relationships. Groups offer an opportunity to focus on these issues and hence shift attention away from the preoccupation with weight and food intake. But it must be emphasised that the group does not offer treatment or therapy. Also the group is not an alternative to therapy. The group offers a regular environment in which many of the issues and problems associated with anorexia or bulimia can be aired and advice and support offered. A most valuable aspect is that the pooling of resources, experience, information, coping strategies, etc., allows participants to feel valued. The activity of helping another person is powerfully reinforcing for the helper. Hence profound changes in thinking and behaviour can occur as a result of group activities.

Self-help strategies

In this chapter so far we have identified a number of positive features of self-help groups which can contribute significantly to the process of recovery. Factors such as reducing feelings of isolation, encouraging a sense of mastery, effectiveness and power in one's life, reducing self-criticism and increasing self-tolerance, etc., all serve to help create a sense of self-identity and encourage autonomy.

In this section we will consider three practical ways of increasing coping ability: relaxation, constructive thinking and problem-solving. These 'coping strategies' or 'self-management techniques', have been shown to be effective methods for dealing with stress and a wide range of emotional difficulties.

1 Relaxation. There are many ways of relaxing and it is advisable for each individual to try various methods in order to find out which are most effective for them. In this section I will outline a method of relaxation that involves three stages: first, inducing relaxation through control of the breath; second, a series of exercises for relaxing the muscles; and, third, relaxing through the use of the imagination. The important thing to note about relaxation is that it is a skill that has to be learned. These exercises need to be practised if they are to work. It may be necessary to practise them every day for two or three weeks before you start to feel their effects.

Stage one: Breathing. Try to set aside 30 minutes when you will not be interrupted, sit in a comfortable armchair, or lie on your bed. Become aware of your breathing. Notice which parts of your body move as you breathe in, and as you breathe out. Notice the speed of your breathing.

Notice if it is your abdomen (or stomach) that moves as you breathe in and out, or if it is your chest region. When you are tense you will probably find that it is the chest area that moves as you breathe in and out. Also when you are tense you will usually find the breath is rapid, or you will tend to hold your breath.

By contrast, when you are relaxed your abdomen will move as you breathe in and out, instead of your chest. When you take a deep breath you will find the abdomen will rise first, and the chest second, as the lungs fill up with air. You can help to relax your breathing by first placing one hand on your abdomen and the other hand on your chest (this is to help you be aware of their movements). As you breathe in, gently move your abdomen out before your chest moves, to encourage the breath to fill the lower part of your lungs first. Notice the movement of your hands. When you are very relaxed your abdomen will rise and fall very gently and your chest will barely move at all.

A relaxed rate of breathing is in the region of 10-12 breaths per minute, although there is naturally some variation between individuals. Try to breathe at a steady pace. It may help to count slowly in your mind as you breathe in and out as follows:

(breathe in)   (breathe out)

one and two ...   and three and four and ...

Each complete breath (in and out) will then last about five or six seconds.

With this first stage the important thing is to find a comfortable relaxed rhythm, so don't force yourself to keep at this pace if you find it feels uncomfortably quick or slow. Try this for a few minutes before going on to the second stage.

Stage two: Muscular relaxation. This part of the relaxation sequence will take about 20 minutes initially, but can be abbreviated as your skill increases. The basic principle of muscular relaxation is to briefly tense a particular muscle group and then release the tension. For each of the ten steps in the relaxation exercise you will tighten your muscles for about ten seconds and then suddenly let go of the tension. Let go of the tension in the muscle at the same time as you breathe out, and at the same time say to yourself 'relax'. Repeat each step twice before going on to the next step.

Fists.	Stretch out both of your arms in front of you and clench both fists. Continue to breathe normally. Be aware of the feeling of tension in your fists. When you breathe out for the third time, suddenly let go of the tension in your fists. As you do this say to yourself: 'Relax'. Notice the difference between the tension and the relaxation.
Forearms.	Stretch out your arms in front of you and point your fingers up to the ceiling with your palms pointing away from you. Continue to breathe normally. Be aware of the feelings of tension in your forearms. When you breathe out for the third time, suddenly let go of the tension in your forearms. As you do this say to yourself: 'Relax'. Notice the difference between the tension and the relaxation.
Biceps.	Try to touch your shoulders with your fists. As you do this clench your bicep muscles tight. Continue to breathe normally. Be aware of the tension in your biceps. When you breathe out for the third time, suddenly

let go of the tension in your biceps. As you do this say to yourself: 'Relax'. Notice the difference between the tension and the relaxation.

Shoulders. Push your shoulders up towards your ears. Continue to breathe normally. Be aware of the feeling of tension in the shoulders, and neck area. When you breathe out for the third time, suddenly let go of the tension in your shoulders. As you do this say to yourself: 'Relax'. Notice the difference between the tension and the relaxation.

Forehead. Just using the muscles of your forehead push your eyebrows up towards your hair, making your brow wrinkle. Continue to breathe normally. Be aware of the feelings of tension in your forehead. When you breathe out for the third time suddenly let go of the tension in your forehead. As you do this say to yourself: 'Relax'. Notice the difference between the tension and the relaxation.

Face. Tense the muscles of your face by closing your eyes tightly, pushing your lips together, clenching your teeth and pushing your tongue to the roof of your mouth. Continue to breathe normally. Be aware of the feelings of tension in your face. When you breathe out for the third time, suddenly let go of the tension in your face. As you do this say to yourself: 'Relax'. Notice the difference between the tension and the relaxation.

Chest. Take in a deep breath, fill your lungs. Hold your breath for five seconds. Be aware of the feelings of tension in your chest area. Then let go of the breath and say to yourself: 'Relax'. Notice the difference between the tension and the relaxation.

Stomach. Tense your stomach muscles making them hard as if you were preparing to receive a blow. At the same time hold your breath for five seconds. Be aware of the feelings of tension in your stomach. Then let go of the tension in your stomach and breathe out. As you do this say to yourself: 'Relax'. Notice the difference between the tension and the relaxation.

Thighs. Tense your thigh muscles by pushing your feet hard against the floor. Continue to breathe normally. Be aware of the feelings of tension in your thighs. When you breathe out for the third time, suddenly let go of the tension in your thigh muscles. As you do this say to yourself: 'Relax'. Notice the difference between the tension and the relaxation.

Calves.   Tense your calf muscles by lifting your feet off the ground and pointing your toes back towards your face. Continue to breathe normally. Be aware of the feelings of tension in your calves. When you breathe out for the third time, suddenly let go of the tension in your calf muscles. As you do this say to yourself: 'Relax'. Notice the difference between the tension and the relaxation.

Stage three: Imagination. The relaxation induced by the breathing and muscle exercises can often be deepened through use of the imagination. One method is to imagine your body becoming deeply relaxed as it sinks deeper into the armchair or bed. As well as picturing this to yourself you can say, in your mind, that you are sinking into the chair, deeply relaxed. You may also have particular natural scenes that you find relaxing, such as lying on a sunny beach, or sitting in a garden. The scene can be one you are familiar with or one you invent. The important thing is to try to conjure up the relaxing scene in as much detail as you can. Imagine not just the appearance, the colours and light and so forth, but also the sounds, the scents, the 'feel' of the place. Allow yourself to become absorbed in this relaxing scene for five minutes or so.

When you rouse yourself from your relaxation do so slowly and quietly, don't immediately start rushing around. After practising these three stages of relaxation a few times you will be able to follow the whole sequence from memory, without having to refer to this book. When you can do this complete all three stages with your eyes closed.

2 Constructive thinking. If we can learn to control our thinking it is possible to significantly reduce the impact of stressful situations. 'Negative feelings' such as despair, sorrow, helplessness, resentment, anger, worthlessness, etc., can all be modified through a process often termed 'cognitive restructuring'. The foundation of this coping strategy is the claim that we create our feelings of distress, or anger, or any other emotional disturbance, through our thinking. This idea was stated long ago by the stoic philosopher Epictetus who wrote: 'Men are disturbed not by things, but by the views which they take of them.' William Shakespeare expressed the same idea in Hamlet: 'There's nothing either good or bad but thinking makes it so.' The way we think will influence what we feel. 'Dysfunctional' thinking will tend to make us experience negative feelings, which disrupt coping ability. Constructive thinking will tend to make us experience positive feelings that encourage coping ability.

We can identify two levels of 'cognitive restructuring'. Level one concerns conscious 'inner mental monologue', or 'self-talk'. This refers to the stream of thoughts which run through the mind virtually non-stop. Level two involves examining and changing both the way in which we interpret events, and the specific beliefs which underlie these interpretations. It is our interpretations and beliefs which give rise to our conscious 'self-talk'.

Level one: 'Cognitive restructuring'. The first step in level one is essentially an exercise in awareness. Next time you experience any emotional disturbance, or face a difficult situation, try to notice what it is you are saying to yourself. As soon as possible try to make a note of the situation and the thoughts which came into your mind. Initially it is difficult to identify this 'self-talk', as these thoughts are often automatic, rapid, and occur without reflection or elaboration. But once you have started to take notice of what it is you are saying to yourself you will find particular themes repeat themselves; you will identify a very personal pattern of private 'self-talk'. You will see that when you experience distress or negative feelings, your self-talk will also be negative. Once you have done this, the next step is to work out positive or constructive patterns of self-talk, which you can use deliberately as an alternative to your habitual patterns of negative thinking.

Below is an example illustrating how this is done. This list is based on one written by Pamela the mother of Helen a 14-year-old anorexic.

> *Situation:* Helen refused to eat anything today; this led to a furious row between Helen and her father.

> **Negative self-talk:**
> 'Doesn't she realise what she's doing to us?'
> 'What did we do wrong?'
> 'Why is this happening to us?'
> 'We used to be so happy, our lives have been ruined.'
> 'Nothing ever goes right.'

'I can't stand this situation any longer.'
'We'll never get over this.'
'Why isn't she like her sister.'
'I'm fed-up with both of them. I wish I could just get up and go.'
'Why hasn't that therapist helped her.'

Positive alternatives:
'Just stay focused on the problem.'
'It won't help blaming ourselves, no-one's to blame.'
'I've coped in the past and I can cope now.'
'The situation is difficult but we are learning to deal with it.'
'We can get through this.'
'Stay calm and relax.'
'Concentrate on what's happening now.'
'We can support each other.'

Donald Meichenbaum, an American psychologist, suggests preparing a series of 'positive self-talk' statements which can be memorised and repeated to oneself before and during stressful situations. These statements need to be focused on actions, and need to be realistic. It will not help if your 'positive self-talk' reflects unobtainable goals or is completely unrealistic. Focus on practical, realistic ways of dealing with the situation.

Two other useful techniques are 'thought-stopping' and 'mental diversion'. Thought-stopping involves identifying unhelpful thoughts or images and immediately stopping them, perhaps by slamming a book on a table and shouting to yourself mentally: **'STOP!'**. Some people find it helpful to picture in their minds a large brightly coloured **'STOP'** sign. This may need to be repeated several times before the negative thoughts stop, but with practice considerable control can be gained over unwanted thoughts. Mental diversion involves distracting yourself by focusing on positive alternative lines of thought. These may be anything which can catch your interest such as hobbies, holidays, and social events. Any form of activity, from listening to music to household chores, can be used as a way of interrupting a negative train of thought.

Level two: 'Cognitive restructuring'. This second level attempts to understand and change (or 'restructure') deeper aspects of negative thinking. Level one 'cognitive restructuring' involves working at a fairly superficial level. Substantial

change in coping ability only really follows from rejecting negative self-talk, not merely avoiding it. That is, negative self-talk
needs to be seen to be false as well as unhelpful. The work of
Albert Ellis, an American psychologist, and the work of Aaron
T. Beck, an American psychiatrist, provide detailed approaches
to cognitive restructuring. Albert Ellis suggests that it is a
person's fundamental beliefs about themselves and the world
that generates emotional disturbance. Beck has identified a
number of thinking errors, or 'cognitive distortions', which
accompany and perhaps lead to 'negative emotions' (such as
depression, anxiety, anger, resentment, etc.). The first step in
level two 'cognitive restructuring' is similar to that of level one
noted above: it is necessary to become aware of the thinking
that accompanies emotional disturbance. When you experience
stress, depression, anxiety, or any other difficult or disruptive
feeling, try to notice exactly what thoughts you have. Beck calls
these 'negative automatic thoughts'. Write these down as precisely as you can. Once you have identified these thoughts the
next step is to analyse them using four questions:

What is the effect of thinking the way I do?
What evidence is there for and against these ideas?
What thinking errors am I making?
What is another way of looking at the situation?

As an example consider once again Helen's row with her
father about her eating.

> One of the 'negative automatic thoughts' identified by Pamela, her
> mother, was 'Our lives have been ruined, we will never get over this.
> I should have done something to prevent this sooner.' This can in
> fact be broken down into three statements or ideas:
> Our lives have been ruined.
> We will never get over this.
> I should have done something to prevent this sooner.

Using this as an example, how could we reply to the four
questions given above? First, **what will be the effects of such
thinking?**

> Pamela made the following list of the feelings and behaviours which
> accompanied and followed her negative thinking:

Feelings:
depressed,
helpless,
demoralised,
without hope,
felt like giving up,
upset,
tearful,
despairing,
wanting to get away from it all.

Behaviour:
withdrew from Helen and Frank,
tried to get away to be on my own,
chain smoked,
cried,
couldn't eat,
left the washing-up,
couldn't sleep.

Pamela's list illustrates the point that negative thinking increases negative feelings, and reduces ability to cope. Becoming aware of such bad effects can provide us with a powerful incentive to work at changing our thought patterns, in order to reduce negative feelings and increase coping ability.

Second, **what evidence is there for and against these ideas?** Consider the evidence for, and against, each negative thought. Is it really the case that the lives of all family members are 'ruined'? What is meant by this? Does it mean that mother, father and daughter, will never feel happiness, satisfaction or pleasure again? Clearly such an extreme claim is unlikely to be true. So does 'ruined' mean not as good as it could be? But even this statement is not true. The only way for the situation to be different now would be if the past had been different. But obviously the past cannot possibly be different. The present cannot be otherwise than it is. All that can be different is the future. And yet this negative thought predicts the future – 'we will never get over this'. So this too is false. Pamela readily acknowledged that she simply did not know what the future would bring. Helen may well recover and the family be brought closer together as a result of the challenge of anorexia nervosa. This certainly happens in some families, and of course Pamela could not be sure that it wouldn't happen in hers. Further, Pamela's self-criticism when she says to herself 'I should have done something sooner', ignores the fact that she had acted in her daughter's best interests given the knowledge she had at the time. Again it is impossible to change the past, and so the most constructive approach is to look to the future and what can be done to improve the situation.

Third, **what thinking errors can we identify?** A list of 'cognitive distortions', or thinking errors based on Beck's work has been given in chapter 3. These disturbances in thinking are certainly not unique to anorexics and bulimics. Any emotional disturbance, or difficulty in coping, will be accompanied by similar thinking errors. Hence parents, spouses, relatives and friends, in trying to help deal with the many difficulties associated with eating disorders, may find themselves engaging in the same kinds of distorted thinking.

In order to help identify thinking errors Beck and his colleague Gary Emery suggest the following questions:

Am I thinking in all-or-nothing terms?
Am I condemning myself as a total person on the basis of a single event?
Am I concentrating on my weaknesses and forgetting my strengths?
Am I blaming myself for something which is not my fault?
Am I taking something personally which has little or nothing to do with me?
Am I expecting myself to be perfect?
Am I using a double standard – how would I view someone else in my situation?
Am I paying attention only to the black side of things?
Am I overestimating the chances of disaster?
Am I exaggerating the importance of events?
Am I fretting about the way things ought to be instead of accepting and dealing with them as they come?
Am I assuming I can do nothing to change my situation?
Am I predicting the future instead of experimenting with it?

Pamela noted her 'negative automatic' thought was an example of dichotomous, or all-or-nothing thinking, catastrophising, and over-generalisation.

Once you can identify the errors involved in your negative thinking you can really work on the fourth question.

Our fourth question concerns looking for alternatives to the 'negative automatic thought'. **What is another way of looking at the situation?** One option would be to resist the tendency to label the situation as a disaster, a 'ruin', and focus on problem-solving. No one doubts that the situation is a difficult one, and that the family face a great challenge. But it is far more helpful to stick with the idea that the situation is difficult, a problem for which solutions can be sought, rather than a completely hopeless disaster. Some aspects of the situation are positive: family members care for each other, helping agencies are involved, Helen is co-operating with therapy, etc. It is important to remember other families have coped in similar situations. Focus on practical problem-solving thoughts and behaviour, rather than imagining the worse. At present we do not know what the future will bring, but whatever happens we will cope better, and respond to the challenge more adaptively, if we stay focused on dealing with practical problems and remain as optimistic as we can.

This section on cognitive restructuring has a very wide application. Working to change distorted, negative thinking into reasonable positive thinking can lead to very dramatic changes in how we feel and act. Very often these techniques are of great value in increasing self-esteem. Low self-esteem is often a central issue for both the anorexic or bulimic sufferer, and those close to her. These cognitive techniques can be very effective in combating feelings of self-criticism, hopelessness, and despair. But they will only work through persistent efforts at identifying and changing negative thinking, and actively cultivating reasonable and positive alternatives.

3 Problem-solving. In addition to relaxation and cognitive restructuring, a systematic approach to problem-solving can be of great value. After analysing our thinking using the four questions noted above, we can ask a fifth question: **What action can I take?** Now it may be the case that you feel you are already doing all you can to improve the situation but it is important to think systematically about your whole range of possible options.

In the approach to problem-solving outlined below there are ten stages:

1 Orientation
2 Define the problem(s)
3 'Brainstorm' solutions
4 Assess feasibility of solutions
5 Specify goals
6 Consider consequences
7 Plan steps to goal
8 Decide
9 Act
10 Evaluate.

Stage one: Orientation. The essential starting point concerns our attitude to our problems. First, it is important to recognise that difficulties are a normal part of life: problems of one sort or another are inevitable. Second, don't underestimate your problem-solving capacity: you have already faced, and dealt effectively, with numerous difficulties in the course of your life. Third, note that problem-solving is a skill than can be improved if we work at applying a systematic approach. And fourthly, try to view problems as challenges, and as opportunities to learn.

Stage two: Define the problem(s). The second stage involves getting a clear statement of the problem(s). In defining the problem you need to be very specific. An initial formulation of a problem may often be quite general, perhaps even vague, and will need to be broken down into more precise statements. A formulation of a specific problem will usually involve a statement which includes two elements: a goal (or desire) and an obstacle. If your formulation, or problem definition, includes more than one goal it is too general and will need to be further subdivided.

For example, Lorna and David were experiencing problems in their marriage; much of the conflict centred around Gill, their 15-year-old anorexic daughter.

Lorna defined the problem as follows: 'David and I are not getting on, we argue all the time. I don't feel he supports me at all, I think we're heading for divorce.'

After some discussion Lorna broke this general statement down into a list of very specific problems, expressed in terms of goals (or desires) and obstacles, all of which contributed to the marriage problem as she saw it. Lorna's list included the following:

'I would like David to spend more time at home in the evening, but he insists he must work late, and then he goes for a drink with his colleagues.'

'David wants Gill to take extra lessons to make sure she doesn't fail her exams. I don't want to put more pressure on her.'

'I am concerned that David is drinking too much, but every time I mention it we get into an argument.'

'David thinks Gill is just being awkward; he wants to force her to eat. I feel if we force her we will make the problem worse.'

Lorna's initial general statement about her marital problem was broken down into 11 precise statements of specific problems each one being a source of conflict and stress. Remember, at this stage your aim is to formulate your problems as precisely as you can. Once you have divided problems into specific areas you can then work on them individually. Start with the easier problems first.

Stage three: 'Brainstorm' solutions. Stage two focused on formulating specific problems in terms of goals (or desires), and obstacles. Solutions to problems usually involve attempting to change our goals, or look for ways to deal with obstacles. During this third stage of problem-solving try to think of as many ways of solving the problem as possible. Ask yourself: 'How can I overcome the obstacles to reach this goal. Or how can I change the goal to one more easily obtainable?' The important point to remember at this stage is that you are trying to list as many alternative solutions as possible – no matter how improbable the alternatives seem. Aim for the maximum number of options, exclude none. This technique is often called 'brainstorming'. It is a way of 'loosening up' your thinking in order to increase the chances of identifying a viable solution that might not be immediately obvious.

> Lorna's 'brainstorming' list of solutions to her conflict with David over whether to force Gill to eat more included the following options:
> 'Try to convince David that I'm right.'
> 'Ignore David.'
> 'Go on holiday and forget about everything.'
> 'Threaten to leave if David doesn't accept my view.'
> 'Accept David's view and let him try to force her to eat.'
> 'Send Gill away to live with her grandmother.'
> 'Make David come to the self-help group so they can tell him.'
> 'Get Gill's therapist to tell him what to do.'

Remember 'brainstorming' is about generating ideas. List every solution that occurs to you even if it is completely impossible.

Stage four: Assess feasibility of solutions. During this stage work through your 'brainstorming' list of solutions and try to assess the feasibility of each option. If you have carried out stage three effectively there will be many 'solutions' that will be impossible to apply. This is as it should be because 'brainstorming' is about generating as many alternatives as possible. During this stage delete from your list all the impractical, or impossible options you have listed. Your aim at this stage is to draw up a list of feasible, or realistic solutions. For each option listed ask yourself: Is this a viable option? Can this be carried out? If you have any doubts about the feasibility of an option don't delete it, keep it on your list for further consideration.

Stage five: Specify goals. You should now have a list of feasible options. These may involve changes in goals (or desires), or changes in your approach to obstacles. Whatever changes your solutions propose the next stage is to express them in terms of specific goals. That is, rewrite them in the form of clear statements which indicate exactly what change is required. When doing this two points need to be borne in mind: first, goals should be realistic; second, as far as possible goals need to be expressed in terms of specific changes in behaviour (i.e. what needs to be done).

> For example, Lorna's list of possible solutions to her conflict with David over Gill's eating included the following option:
> 'Get Gill's therapist to tell David what to do.'
> Lorna rewrote this option in the form of a specific goal that was both realistic and focused on changes in behaviour. Lorna specified her goal as follows:
> 'Arrange a meeting where David, myself, and Gill's therapist can discuss this conflict together.'

Stage six: Consider consequences. This is often the hardest part of the problem-solving strategy, and at first sight can seem laborious. But if it is carried out with care it can greatly clarify thinking and reduce the difficulty of decision-making. During this stage you need to think through the consequences of each of the alternatives generated through the 'brainstorming' exercise that remain on your list after completing stage four (assessing feasibility). This stage comprises three steps. First, divide consequences into 'short-term' (i.e. what will immediately happen if you carry out the option), and 'long-term' (i.e. what will be the result, days, weeks, or months later). Second, look through your list of short-term and long-term consequences, and label each one positive or negative. After carrying out these two steps you will be able to make a list for each option using the following outline:

Consequences (option 1)

	short-term	long-term
Positives	1	....
	2	....
	3	....
	etc.	
Negatives	1	....
	2	....
	3	....
	etc.	

Once this has been done we can go on to the third step. A judgment needs to be made as to the **overall** short-term and long-term consequences. That is, you need to look through your list of short-term consequences and decide whether, as a whole and on balance, they are positive or negative. The same needs to be done for the long-term consequences. For each solution there are four possible outcomes:

	short-term	long-term
outcome 1	positive	positive
outcome 2	negative	positive
outcome 3	positive	negative
outcome 4	negative	negative

As a general guide the order of preference would be as listed here. That is, outcome one (positive short-term and positive long-term consequences) is the best option. Outcome two, is second best, and so on. A common error is to opt for a solution with a positive-negative outcome (outcome three) when we have no clear positive-positive (outcome one) solution. This is because of the immediate short-term benefits of outcome three. But in general outcome two (negative-positive) will usually be a better choice than outcome three (positive-negative).

Lorna felt the option of setting up a meeting between herself, Gill's therapist and David, to discuss their conflict would probably have negative short-term consequences as David might well resent Lorna's appeal to an authority outside the home. However, she felt such a discussion would be very likely to have positive long-term consequences as she felt sure David would be able to communicate with and respond to the therapist.

Stage seven: Plan steps to goal. Stage seven of problem-solving involves thinking of the steps that will need to be taken to accomplish your specified goal. Make sure each step you list is a concrete approach to your goal. Some of these may involve dealing with obstacles, which may be regarded as sub-goals. Keep each step as simple as possible, and specify the task in terms of what you need to do. For example, Lorna's steps included:

'Contact Gill's therapist to discuss possibility of arranging a meeting.'
'Ask Gill's therapist for suggestions of how to approach David with the request that he attends the appointment.'
'Discuss the difficulty at the self-help group and listen to their suggestions.'
'Discuss the conflict with my therapist and ask for further suggestions.'

Stage eight: Decide. You are now in a position to consider your decision. The best option(s), or solution(s) you have, are those with outcomes one or two (i.e. where consequences are positive-positive, or negative-positive). If you have an option with a negative-positive outcome, and an option with a positive-negative outcome (i.e. outcome three) resist the temptation to go for the latter and stick with the former. Make use of the order for outcome preference (stage six above), as a guide to decision-making.

Stage nine: Act. Once you have spent time systematically examining your possible solutions, and have made a decision, the next stage is to follow through with action. You will need to persist with the option you have decided to take unless new information causes you to reappraise the feasibility, or the consequences, of your choice.

Stage ten: Evaluation. It is useful to keep the notes you make in the course of thinking through these stages of problem-solving. Once you have embarked on a course of action make sure you regularly review the goals and tasks you have set yourself. If new problems arise it may be because the steps towards a goal were not thought out in sufficient detail, or perhaps the goal will need revising. Look back through your notes when you evaluate progress and repeat stages as necessary.

This procedure may appear long-winded at first sight, but through practice you will find greater confidence in dealing with problems, and become more efficient at finding solutions.

8 Providing support

Anorexics, bulimics and their families, often come into contact with a wide range of professional and voluntary workers who can be of great help in assisting the process of recovery. Nurses, nursing assistants, occupational therapists, dieticians and teachers, as well as people involved in voluntary or self-help organisations, will often spend more time with a person suffering from an eating disorder, and their families, than the sufferer's doctor or therapist. This chapter outlines the essential characteristics of helping or supportive relationships. The general approach outlined here is derived from studies of helping relationships in general. The material in this chapter is applicable to any relationship in which one person is trying to offer help to another person who is experiencing difficulties in their life. The principles outlined in this chapter will provide a framework for offering support to anorexics, bulimics and their families. Support may be provided during a single interaction, or it may be a feature of an ongoing relationship. In both cases the principles discussed in this chapter will apply. The suggestions in this chapter will help you create the conditions that will encourage communication, but it should be borne in mind that anorexia and bulimia are characterised by disturbances in thinking and perception which often make communication difficult. The list of 'cognitive distortions' given in chapter 3, and the suggestions for communication in chapters 5 and 6 will help you anticipate some of the difficulties that may arise.

To begin let us be clear about what is meant by 'providing support'. We are concerned with creating a relationship, or an interaction, in which the other person feels safe, accepted, valued, and free to talk about and be herself. We may define 'support' as: the provision of encouragement, the enhancement of morale, and the maintenance of sociability, together with specific practical assistance. Anorexics and bulimics often experience their relationships to be the opposite of this, being characterised by: misunderstanding, threat, dismissal, and rejection. A genuine, supportive relationship can be a powerful factor in preventing withdrawal, isolation, and demoralisation. For someone with an eating disorder this can be a very significant factor in the process of recovery.

This chapter will discuss how such a supportive relationship can be developed. It may be noted that genuine friendship will provide such support, as it were, 'naturally'. Some might argue it is somewhat artificial, or even insincere, to try to study 'how to do it'. However a great deal of our behaviour in relationships is a product of learning, even much of our behaviour that we usually term 'natural'. Whether you are supportive or unsupportive in your relationships you are so largely as a result of what you have learned. This chapter is based on the premise that if you desire to help or support someone who is experiencing difficulties in their life you can benefit from learning some of the principles of how such support can be provided. If you try some of these suggestions you may initially feel a little awkward. But if you continue to make use of them this feeling will pass and they will become part of your natural way of interacting.

If we want to offer support to another person the first indispensable step is to examine ourselves. If we can accept and value ourselves, then we can accept and value others. The extent to which we can be open to our own difficult feelings – without reacting with fear, criticism or judgement – will influence the extent to which we can be exposed to the distress or turmoil of another person and respond sensitively. In addition to examining how we feel about ourselves, we need to be aware of how we feel about other people. If we view other people positively, if we value them, it will be much easier to respond to them in helpful ways. This chapter deals with various 'relationship skills' which will indicate how support can be provided in a relationship. However, it is important to realise that our feelings about ourselves and others emerge in our interactions, and no amount of practice in 'relationship skills' will cover, or compensate for, our personal feelings and attitudes. As an example, assume you are in contact with the mother of an anorexic teenager. If you believe parents, especially mothers, are to blame for their daughter's illness, and assume you also have strong feelings of resentment towards your own mother, responding in helpful ways to this mother's distress will be very difficult indeed.

Given that the most significant factor in providing support is your own feelings about yourself and the other person, there are a number of skills that can be learned through practice that can facilitate the growth of a supportive relationship. The rest of this chapter will focus on these skills.

Listening

Respecting the other person's experience. The experience of really being listened to, of really being heard, seems to be very rare. Often people may appear to be listening, but their thoughts are elsewhere. How often have you said something to someone and later realised they have either not heard, or you have been misunderstood? To really listen to another person is to take them seriously. It is a powerful form of affirmation. Genuine careful listening requires deep respect for the other person's experience. If your underlying attitude is that someone with an eating disorder is either being 'silly' or 'awkward', that is if you tend to dismiss her or blame her, you will not be able to listen to her, you will not hear what she says – if indeed she says anything to you. By really listening to another person you affirm them. You may believe that what they say is mistaken or exaggerated as in the 'cognitive distortions' discussed in chapter 3. But in order to really listen the essential factor is not agreement with what is said, but respect for the thoughts, feelings and experience of the other person. Respect for the experience of the other person is the best foundation from which to try to understand that experience.

Verbal, vocal, and non-verbal communication. Careful listening involves giving attention to what is said, how it is said, and what is being communicated non-verbally. These three, the verbal, vocal, and non-verbal communications may not all be 'saying' the same thing. For example if a verbal communication said: 'I'm not upset', but the voice quivered (vocal communication), and the person's eyes remained lowered so you could not engage in eye contact (non-verbal communication), you would probably be correct to assume the opposite of the verbal communication. A good listener will pay attention to these three forms of communication and will attempt to understand all three. It is important to remember that people do not always say what they mean, and one may need to do a lot of translating, or decoding, in order to understand what is being communicated. Below is a list of areas of significant non-verbal communications. However it must be emphasised that there are no fixed rules which allow us to give precise meanings to particular non-verbal behaviours. The meaning of non-verbal communication varies enormously depending on the situation in which it occurs, the nature of the relationship, and the cultural background of the people involved. Hence interpretations of the meaning of non-verbal communication must always be tentative. Your non-verbal communication will be sending messages continually, and can, in themselves, be supportive and reassuring. It is important to bear in mind that in addition to being attentive to the other person's non-verbal communication you need to be aware of what your 'body language' is saying. Good listening involves attending to the other person in such a way that you convey your attention, interest, and respect.

1 **Physical availability**. How available is the other person for you, and how available are you for them? Availability here refers to how often you see and talk to each other. There may be many reasons why one person avoids seeing another person, but often avoidance will be interpreted as rejection. In order to be genuinely supportive you need to be available. Further, being physically available needs to be a reliable feature of your relationship.

2 **Physical proximity**. The amount of 'personal space' felt to be appropriate between two people will depend on a number of factors including the type of relationship they have, what they are discussing, and their cultural background. Be aware of the distance between you and the other person, notice how comfortable you feel. Moving closer can be experienced by someone as very supportive, or it can be experienced as threatening. If someone moves away from you during an interaction it may indicate withdrawal or discomfort. If they move away just after you move closer you may have invaded their 'personal space' and you will need to take careful note of this. Leaning forward can be a simple way of conveying interest and attentiveness.

3 **Physical contact**. Physical contact, for example, putting your arm around someone, can be experienced in many ways. It can have many meanings. In some contexts it can be very supportive and reassuring. In others it may be seen as intrusive and even

threatening. It may be valued as a warm friendly gesture, or rejected as an unwanted sexual advance. Physical contact in our society is surrounded by a great many rules. It is very easy for misunderstandings to occur. However, there is no doubt that appropriate physical contact, even if it is simply a light touch on someone's arm, can be experienced as enormously supportive and helpful.

4 **Physical orientation**. Physical orientation refers to the angle at which you place yourself in relation to another person. In order to interact well with someone you will need to be able to have eye contact, and be able to observe non-verbal communication. Also you will want them to be able to see your non-verbal communication and responses. However, facing another person head on is probably not very helpful. This position can easily be experienced as threatening, or too closed in. Very often a more comfortable position for both parties, is to be at a slight angle to each other, so that you need to turn your head slightly in order to see each other. This orientation allows more 'space' to the other person, and is much less likely to be experienced as a confrontation.

5 **Body posture**. Body posture is a useful indication of a person's emotional availability. Sitting with legs and arms crossed, back erect and staring at the floor indicate closure. This posture will usually mean the person does not want to open up and interact. Although they are communicating a very powerful message (i.e. leave me alone!) they are likely to be resistant to entering into any other communication. If you approach another person with an open, relaxed posture, you are more likely to put them at ease and demonstrate that you are emotionally available. It is reassuring to others if you are relaxed, but sloppiness is likely to be irritating.

6 **Physical appearance**. Through our appearance we say a great deal about ourselves. Of course a change in physical appearance is the most obvious symptom of anorexia nervosa. But appearance can tell us much more than simply that someone is starving. A person experiencing extreme stress, or depression, may neglect their appearance. This may be very startling if it occurs where someone had previously been very careful about their appearance. But even small changes can be significant and may be a sign that the person is having difficulty coping.

7 **Gestures**. Gestures can be used to emphasise what you have said, and to express feelings. If you are talking with a friend who assures you they are not annoyed but you notice they have clenched their fist, you will probably be correct to be sceptical about their verbal communication, and put more weight on what is being communicated non-verbally. Simple gestures can convey

powerful messages. A hand raised, palm towards you even if briefly, may indicate a desire to push you away, or shut you up. Be aware of these communications and adapt your response accordingly.

8 **Head and body movement**. Movement can indicate interest, or animation, or it can signal boredom or irritation. In order to interpret these communications correctly you will need to observe facial expression, and eye contact in particular, to see what message they contain. When you speak be aware that moving can show interest and engagement in the conversation but make sure your movements are appropriate to what you are saying. Body movements that need to be avoided include tapping your fingers or foot, or any mannerisms that can be a distraction. Head nods are important indicators of interest or agreement, and are usually experienced as rewarding. However, head nods can signal impatience, so once again it is important to look carefully at the whole range of non-verbal behaviours in order to understand what is being communicated.

9 **Facial expression**. The richest source of non-verbal communication is probably the facial area. A smile is the most immediate and obvious indication of friendliness and interest. Small movement of the eyebrows can indicate concentration, interest, surprise, and even disbelief. It is, of course, essential that facial expression matches the verbal communication of yourself or the other person. Smiling when someone is in distress will destroy any feelings of warmth or support in the relationship. Observe someone's face during an interaction and you will notice the changes occurring in the course of the conversation. These changes in facial expression can tell you a great deal about the changing feelings and responses of other people.

10 **Eye contact**. Eye contact is a vital part of non-verbal communication. Generally people in a conversation 'take turns' looking directly at each other's eyes. The person talking will usually look away from the listener's eyes, while the listener will look at the face and eyes of the speaker. Someone who never looks directly at your eyes, even when they are speaking, may be very anxious or depressed ,or even angry. This lack of eye contact will represent a barrier between you and the other person that will need to be responded to with care if it is to be overcome.

In addition to paying careful attention to verbal, vocal and non-verbal communication, good listening involves inhibiting responses which we may be tempted to make, but which are in fact far from helpful. The following list has been adapted from that provided by Richard Nelson-Jones, a British psychologist working in Australia, in his book *Human Relationship Skills*.

1 **Directing and leading**. Taking control of what the other person can talk about.
> 'I would like you to talk about your relationship with your mother.'
> 'I would like to know how much you weigh.'
> 'Let's talk about your bingeing and vomiting.'

2 **Judging and evaluating**. Making evaluative statements, especially those that indicate that the other is falling short of your own standards.
> 'You've made a real mess of your life.'
> 'You can't go on like this, you must eat more.'
> 'I'm sure you can do better than that.'

3 **Blaming**. Assigning responsibility for what happens to another in a finger-pointing way.
> 'You've really upset your family.'
> 'I think she's lost weight because of you.'
> 'You've made her worse.'

4 **Getting aggressive**. Making statements that are designed to cause pain and put the other person down.
> 'Look how thin you are, you look terrible.'
> 'You must realise how disgusting it is to binge and vomit.'
> 'It's a waste of time talking to you.'

5 **Moralising and preaching**. Patronisingly telling another person how they should be leading their life.
> 'You should do what your parents tell you.'
> 'You should be grateful for all the help you've received.'
> 'This isn't good enough, you really must get control of her.'

6 **Advising and teaching**. Not giving the other space to arrive at their own solutions to their concerns. Appearing to know best how they should lead their lives.
> 'No wonder you are lonely, you should go out and meet people.'
> 'My advice to you is, eat just a little bit more and you'll be all right.'
> 'Instead of starving yourself you should stand up for yourself.'

7 **Not accepting another's feelings**. Telling people that their feelings should be different from what they are.
> 'I'm sure you don't really feel like that.'
> 'You can't be unhappy, look at all you've got, such a lovely home, and family.'
> 'There's no reason to feel depressed, you're just tired.'

8 **Inappropriately talking about yourself**. Talking about yourself in ways that interfere with another's disclosures.

'I know exactly how you feel, let me tell you about my bingeing.'

'Let me tell you what happened to me, you may learn something from it.'

'I was anorexic once, let me tell you how I got over it.'

9 **Interrogating**. Using questions in such a way that the other feels threatened by unwanted probing.

'How often do you binge?'

'What exactly did you eat?'

'What's your present weight?'

10 **Reassuring and humouring**. Trying to make others feel better more for your sake than theirs. Not really acknowledging their true feelings.

'We all feel like that sometimes.'

'Look, I've made you laugh. It can't be that bad.'

'Lots of people get over anorexia and bulimia.'

11 **Labelling and diagnosing**. Playing the amateur psychologist and placing a label or diagnostic category on another.

'You're a real neurotic.'

'I think you're anorexic.'

'I know what's wrong with you – you've got bulimia.'

12 **Over-interpreting**. Offering explanations for others' behaviour which bear little relationship to what they may have thought of by themselves.

'I think you're not eating because you're afraid to grow up.'

'When you reject food you are rejecting your mother.'

'By vomiting you are trying to get rid of unwanted feelings.'

13 **Distracting and being irrelevant**. Confusing the issue by going off in another direction or creating a smokescreen.

'Families always have problems with teenage daughters, don't worry about it.'

'Talking about this won't help, tell me about your school work.'

'What do you want to do when you've got over this anorexia.'

14 **Faking attention**. Insincerely pretending to be more interested and involved in what is being said than you are.

'How interesting.'

'Oh, really?'

'Is that so?'

15 **Placing time pressures**. Letting the other know that your availability for listening is very limited.

'I'm so busy at the moment.'

'I really must go.'

'I can spend a few minutes talking, but that's all.'

Responding

A good listener will be responding effectively even before they have said a word. A good listener will send a clear message: I am interested in, and value, what you are thinking and feeling. In the previous section we noted how this may be done through non-verbal communication, and through what is not said. In this section we will discuss verbal communication, and how this can contribute to establishing a safe and accepting relationship, which will be experienced as supportive and encouraging. We will consider two forms of verbal response: questions and reflection.

Questions. Questions are an essential means of starting and maintaining an interaction. But there are pitfalls. The following list describes some of the ways questions can actually discourage rather than encourage conversation.

1 **Closed questions.** Closed questions can be answered with one word, like yes or no, and therefore limit possible response options. Open questions require more elaborate replies and therefore invite more extensive interaction. 'Do you want to go for a walk?' is a closed question. 'How do you feel about a walk?' is open. Of course if someone really does not want to talk they can reply to virtually any question with just a few words. But your goal is not to force someone into a conversation, but to invite them or encourage them, to talk. This may be done through asking questions that provide an opportunity for a more elaborate reply than simply one or two words.

2 **Leading questions.** Leading questions involve making a statement for the other person. Such questions put words into the other person's mouth. Some examples of leading questions are: 'You prefer eating out don't you?', 'You will have another piece of cake, won't you?'

3 **Intrusive questions.** Questions of an intimate nature can very easily be experienced as intrusive, and will tend to make the other become defensive and withdraw. It must be appreciated that questions addressed to an anorexic or bulimic about her food intake or weight, will be regarded as an encroachment on their personal life. Such questions are likely to be regarded as every bit as personal as questions about sexual interests or sexual activities. Questions about such private matters will not lead to a supportive and encouraging exchange unless they occur within a relationship that is already characterised by trust, acceptance, warmth and support.

4 **Too many questions**. It is essential that asking questions is not overdone. Asking questions can easily slip into interrogation. Often this occurs because a large number of closed questions are 'fired' at the other person. A person is more likely to engage if they are given the opportunity and space to formulate a reply to an open question. Giving space includes allowing time for the other person to think over their reply without rushing in to fill the silence with more questions.

In contrast to the above there are some questions that can be very useful in opening up channels of communication and encouraging the other person to enter into conversation.

1 **Ask for information**. Asking someone for specific information about something is probably the most straightforward form of questioning. It is relatively easy to ask for specific details, such as: 'What exactly did he say?' 'When did that happen?' 'How long did that go on for?' It will often be easy to generate many of these sorts of questions, but remember that the goal is not for you to get an exact description of an event, but for a supportive interaction to take place. Asking for specific details can facilitate this if used carefully. You do not want to swamp the interaction with facts, so use these questions sparingly.

2 **Ask for elaboration**. These questions invite the speaker to extend, or elaborate on, what has been said. Such questions demonstrate your attentiveness and interest, but be very careful not to become intrusive. You may ask for elaboration simply by saying: 'Can you say more?' or 'Was there anything else?' You can effectively ask for elaboration simply by reflecting back some of the words used by the other person with a questioning tone in your voice. For example, an anorexic told me her feelings had been 'torn out' of her. I repeated the key words as a question: 'Torn out?' She then went on to amplify and elaborate on what she had said.

3 **Ask for clarification**. Questions which express your desire to understand what is said may acknowledge your lack of understanding and request clarification. Examples include questions such as: 'I'm not sure I understand you, could you repeat what you've said?' or 'Can you say that again for me?'

4 **Ask about feelings**. Requests for information, elaboration, or clarification, can often end up focusing conversation on factual details of a situation. This may be helpful, but it can be a means of avoiding more central issues connected with what a person is feeling. Focusing on feelings is an important way of acknowledg-

ing the other person. You can ask about feelings by saying: 'How do you feel about ... ?' or 'What are your feelings about that?' or 'What are you feeling now?'

Questions can be an essential means of facilitating a supportive interaction with another person. However, once again it is important to note that questions should not be over-used. It is sometimes very much more supportive simply to be with someone without saying anything. Do not be afraid of silence. Although silence can be uncomfortable or even threatening, notice how the other person responds non-verbally. At the right time, just being with another person, in silence, can send a powerful message of care and support.

Reflection. In addition to asking questions a very valuable way of encouraging communication and facilitating understanding is the process of 'reflection'. American psychologist Carl Rogers wrote extensively about this in his articles and books on counselling. It is a method of responding to another person that can be an extremely effective way of conveying your concern and interest. However, it is also very easy to misuse, hence very considerable care needs to be taken if you are to attempt to use this way of responding in your relationship.

1 **Reflecting meaning**. The basic principle of reflection is to put back to the person what you understand them to be saying. There are various ways of doing this. You may summarise or paraphrase what is said, perhaps prefacing your summary with: 'Let me make sure I've understood you, you're saying ... ', or, 'So you're saying ...'. You may reflect back some of the exact words used by the other person, especially if the words or images are particularly vivid (as was the case in the example given above of an anorexic who referred to her feelings as being 'torn out' of her). Reflection may be given as a question rather than a restatement of what has been said. For example: 'Have I got this right ... ?' 'Do you mean ... ?' 'Are you saying ... ?'

Reflecting meaning allows you to check that you have understood what has been communicated to you, and for the other person to correct you. But, more importantly, this process also allows the other person to clarify the meanings implicit in what they have said, but are perhaps not fully aware of.

2 **Reflecting feelings**. Some counsellors and therapists who employ reflection in their work suggest that you should not go beyond

what is actually given, or presented, by a speaker. However, that restriction is extremely difficult to sustain and, for all but the most proficient in this approach, the result is often to discourage communication and convey lack of genuine interest and understanding. The creation of a trusting and supportive relationship will be helped by the acknowledgement of the other person's feelings, even if we find these feelings disturbing. Reflecting feelings will often go beyond what is verbally communicated, and will attempt to translate or decode, the vocal and non-verbal communications. Someone may verbally deny they feel upset but their vocal and non-verbal communication will convey their feelings. Reflecting feelings involves conveying your perceptions of what the other person is feeling. Sometimes their feelings will seem obvious, at other times you will clearly be guessing. But it is important not to assume you know how the other person feels. When you reflect back feelings you will often be making a guess at how the person feels, hence don't feel you have to conceal your uncertainty. Also it is worth remembering that it may be less threatening to frame your reflections in terms of statements rather than questions. For example, you may begin your statement by saying: 'I wonder if ... ', or 'I guess you may feel ... ' That is, you convey tentativeness. You are not suggesting you know what the other person is feeling. Your response will be helpful if the other person feels you want to understand, respect, and accept their feelings. If they experience your interaction as one in which their feelings are acknowledged and valued, and not criticised or dismissed, then they will feel supported.

Practical assistance

We have defined support as 'the provision of encouragement, the enhancement of morale, and the maintenance of sociability, together with specific practical assistance.' So far we have discussed the two central features of any interaction: listening and responding. By careful listening and sensitive responding it is possible to create an exchange that will be experienced as rewarding and encouraging, and that will tend to counter demoralisation. If relationships are rewarding people do not withdraw, hence sociability is maintained. However, important as good communication is, there may also be areas of practical assistance which can be offered. Such practical assistance can take many forms from helping someone fill in a job application to accompanying them to a self-help group. However, it is very important that you do not try to solve the other person's problems for them. In the last section of chapter 7 there is an outline for a basic approach to problem-solving. Now in some situations it may be helpful to discuss this approach with someone who is experiencing difficulties. But if this is done you must be sure to let the person use the approach to find their own solutions, and not impose your preferences on them.

Through genuine listening and sensitive responding you will often help the other person to clarify their difficulties and their feelings. In the course of conversation you can both think through possible solutions to difficulties, perhaps employing the approach to problem-solving described in chapter 7. But you must be very careful not to take on the problem yourself. You may help clarify goals, and possible solutions, but the problem as well as the solution remains with the other person.

Summary

This chapter has focused on how to offer support to someone who is experiencing difficulties in their life. The suggestions given here are general and apply to any relationship in which one person is trying to help and support another. By following the suggestions offered in this chapter professionals and voluntary workers will find they will be able to provide encouragement and support to anorexics, bulimics, and their families, through their contacts with them. In the case of an anorexic or a bulimic they will, of course, not be 'cured' as a result. But support, especially through difficult times, is a valuable contribution to the process of recovery.

9 Therapy and outcome

Therapy

What is the most effective treatment for anorexia and bulimia? Unfortunately the answer to this question is: We do not know. There are now many types of treatment, or therapy (I will use these terms interchangeably) available, most of which have not been evaluated. The outcome studies which have been done involve a very restricted range of therapies and in most cases do not look at outcome in the long term. The research base on which to judge competing therapies is therefore very inadequate. There are many difficulties with carrying out research into the effectiveness of various therapies, and a great deal of work still needs to be done. This chapter will outline some of the more widely available approaches to treatment and reference to outcome research will be included in each section. However, there are some important general points to be made before considering specific approaches. First, although some anorexics and bulimics recover without therapy, as a general rule some form of therapy will be necessary. Second, therapy is most effective in the early stages of an eating disorder. Third, although some forms of therapy are more effective than others, there is, as yet, no clear evidence demonstrating the consistent superiority of any one approach. Fourth, different forms of therapy may be more or less effective at different stages of the illness, and with different ages of the sufferer.

Doubtlessly the obvious need for therapeutic help, and the failure of research to demonstrate the superiority of one particular approach has contributed to the proliferation of treatments in this field. However, another important reason is the continuing disagreement about the causes of anorexia and bulimia. Different beliefs about the cause of an eating disorder will give rise to different beliefs about how they should be treated. The model presented in this book, of anorexia and bulimia as conditions with multiple determinants, tries to do justice to a wide range of research evidence and theoretical work on aetiology. But within this general model there is still considerable scope for disagreement. In particular the degree of significance attached to any specific contributing cause will be a matter of dispute.

One major disagreement among therapists concerns the extent to which the distinctive characteristics of anorexia are due to the effects of starvation. Therapists from widely differing backgrounds will agree that starvation has a significant impact on functioning but may disagree about the extent to which the specific thinking, feeling and behaviour of an anorexic can be accounted for by this factor. If a therapist believes much if not all of the 'psychopathology' of anorexia derives from starvation, then obtaining a weight close to that expected for an individual's sex, age and height will be an absolute priority. If this therapist accepts that conflicts regarding, for example, issues of control, are also significant determinants of anorexia these may be addressed but only after restoration of normal weight, which is given priority in treatment because weight loss, or starvation, is given priority as a causal explanation. However, a second therapist may feel the effects of starvation have been exaggerated by our first therapist and will leave questions of food intake and weight and focus instead on the personal issues which are assumed to be the more significant causal factors. There are, then, various approaches to therapy that will be associated with differing opinions about the causes of the conditions. From the view of anorexia and bulimia as conditions with multiple determinants it would follow that a range of therapy options may be employed in an attempt to address the various contributing factors. Hence, a number of the therapies listed in this chapter may be used either concurrently, or at different stages of the illness.

Before outlining the major therapies available in Britain let us be clear on what it is that therapy aims to accomplish. We have seen, in chapter 2, that diagnosis largely centres on two factors. First, there are particular behavioural characteristics: food restriction and weight loss, bingeing and purging. Second, there is a distinctive attitude characterising both anorexia and bulimia. Therapy will aim to address both of these factors, but may do so in different ways. Most therapists would probably agree that for therapy to be successful, that is for the individual to genuinely relinquish her anorexic or bulimic position, weight restoration or managing to prevent the binge-purge cycle is not enough. This is often the easier part of therapy, at least in the short term. The difficult part of therapy, and what is absolutely essential if therapy is to be successful and relapse prevented, is the changing of the 'anorexic attitude'.

Available therapies

Hospitalisation. Under the provisions of the 1983 Mental Health Act compulsory hospitalisation may occur if there is judged to be a serious risk to life. Anorexics and bulimics have been brought into hospital because of the risk of suicide. Also both conditions can lead to life-threatening physical complications. In the case of anorexia a weight 60% of average expected body weight is likely to be regarded as an indication for admission. If an anorexic is at a higher weight but her weight is falling rapidly admission may also be recommended. In all of these cases the individual can be taken into hospital against their will. Voluntary admission may occur in the case of anorexia and bulimia if out-patient or day-patient treatment has not been successful. Hospitalisation for anorexia is very much more common than for bulimia. Hospitalisation does have the advantage of allowing thorough medical examination to exclude other causes of weight loss, and to check what the physical impact of food restriction, or bingeing and purging has been. Admission may be to a medical ward, a psychiatric ward, or to a specialist unit. While in hospital a number of treatments may be offered.

Weight restoration. A number of methods of weight restoration are employed in hospitals. In cases of emergency intravenous feeding may be necessary. In some hospitals nasogastric tubes may be used. Generally the patient will be encouraged to accept a high calorie diet, often started in liquid form. The usual goal will be between 2,000 and 5,000 calories per day, with a weight increase of 3 to 4 lbs per week. The period of hospitalisation will often be two to three months, until weight is at least 90% of average expected body weight. Discharge will usually occur about three to four weeks after this target weight is reached.

Behaviour modification. Hospitals will often employ principles of behaviour modification in the process of weight restoration. The basic principle is to make access to various amenities and 'privileges' dependent on weight gain. The anorexic may be confined to her room without access to radio, television, books, newspapers, phone calls, visitors, perhaps even pillows. She may also not be allowed to leave the room to go to the toilet or the bathroom. She will have to use a commode and wash in the sink. Gradually 'privileges' are restored as weight is increased. The theoretical justification for behaviour modification involves the claim that almost all behaviour is learned, and is primarily determined by the environment. In this context the central idea is that the likelihood of a behaviour being repeated is increased if it is followed by some form of reward, i.e. if it is reinforced. In this case eating and weight gain are rewarded, or reinforced, by restoration of privileges. In the short term, that is while the patient is in hospital, these programmes are very effective in producing weight gain. However, after discharge from hospital the increased weight is very frequently lost. Advocates of the approach say the relapse is because the patient has returned to an environment that does not reward eating and weight gain. However, research suggests many anorexics comply while in hospital just to get out, and are very critical of this approach. It is often argued that to further reduce an anorexic's feeling of control by such a regime is counter-productive and will exacerbate the sense of ineffectiveness which seems to be such a central feature of the condition. This is a very important consideration, and research does support the claim that behaviour modification without psychotherapy or counselling is unlikely to be of benefit to the sufferer in the long term.

Medication. Four classes of drugs have been used in the treatment of anorexia. Major tranquillisers, such as chlorpromazine, may be used with in-patients to reduce anxiety during weight restoration. Minor tranquillisers, such as diazepam, have been used to reduce anxiety, mainly with out-patients. Drugs with appetite-stimulating properties, such as cyprohetadine, have also been used in an attempt to increase the anorexic's food intake. Anti-depressants may be prescribed where there are judged to be significant symptoms of depression. Some doctors believe both anorexia and bulimia are variants of a major depressive disorder. If this is accepted, use of anti-depressants will form the central therapeutic strategy. In the case of anorexia, amitryptaline is the most commonly pre-scribed anti-depressant. Anti-depressants may also be used in the treatment of bulimia, especially imipramine and phenelzine. However, research has shown very modest gains from the use of medication in the treatment of anorexia and bulimia and, in general, medication will tend only to be used as part of a wider approach which includes some form of psychotherapy.

Group therapy. There are many forms of group therapy, and there are many settings in which it may be offered. In-patient, day-patient and out-patient facilities may include some form of group therapy. Group membership may be restricted to those with anorexia or bulimia, or may include patients with various medical or psychiatric problems. Reports suggest the most helpful type of group approach is that which focuses on specific problem-solving tasks, such as developing social skills or deal-ing with interpersonal conflict. Advocates of this approach argue that anorexia and bulimia are maintained by restricted social activity and low self-esteem, difficulties which group work can help to overcome. There is little outcome research on group therapy, but one recent study examining group and individual approaches using cognitive-behaviour therapy (see below) found individual therapy to be more effective.

Family therapy. Family therapists consider the family context to be the crucial factor in the maintenance of an eating disorder. Most of the published work has concerned anorexia rather than bulimia, but similar principles and a similar approach would apply to both. The focus of therapy is what is happening in the family as a whole, rather than the behaviour of the anorexic or the bulimic in isolation. The family will display specific pat-terns of interaction within its own network of relationships. The therapist will seek to identify the role or function that the eating disorder has within this complex pattern of relationships and interactions. The goal of therapy is to discover ways in which particular aspects of family behaviour and communication can be adjusted in order to provide a context in which the eating dis-order can be given up. Initially outcome research reported on families with an anorexic in her very early teens, or even younger, in the early stage of the disorder. Outcome with this client group was reported to be very good, in fact superior to success rates reported in studies of individual therapy. However, critics have pointed out that a young client in the early stages of anorexia was more likely to respond to therapy regardless of whether it is family or individual therapy. In order to compare treatments clients must be matched for age and duration of the disorder. One recent study involved anorexics whose disorder began before they were 19-years-old, and was of less than three years duration. These clients were given either outpatient family therapy, or individual 'supportive' psychotherapy. The family therapy was shown to be markedly superior.

Psychodynamic psychotherapy. There are a number of approaches we can term 'psychodynamic'. These range from classical psychoanalysis, which would involve several sessions a week for many years with an analyst outside the National Health Service, to weekly therapy for a year or two with a psychodynamically orientated psychotherapist in the NHS. The assumption in this approach is that the symptoms of anorexia or bulimia are related to unconscious conflicts, which the therapist will attempt to uncover. Many influential writers in this field have expressed reservations about using classical analysis with anorexics or bulimics. For example, Hilde Bruch wrote: (therapies) 'where the patient expresses his secret thoughts and feelings and the analyst interprets their unconscious meaning, contains for patients with eating disorders elements that represent painful repetition of a pattern that had characterised their whole development, namely of being told by someone else what they think and feel, with the implication that they are incapable of doing it themselves. The profound sense of ineffectiveness that has troubled them all their lives is thus confirmed.' It is certainly true that psychodynamic work can initially make the patient feel less in control and hence may well be experienced as too threatening by those suffering from anorexia or bulimia in which issues of control and self-identity are so important. However, there are reports of the successful use of psychodynamic therapy with anorexics and bulimics, so it would be unwise to rule out this approach completely. It may be that psychodynamic work has value in consolidating and extending improvements which have been secured by other means.

Cognitive-behaviour therapy. This type of therapy may be offered to in-patients, but is more likely to be provided through hospital out-patient services, or health centres. Cognitive-behaviour therapy starts from the assumption that recovery will require changes in both behaviour and thinking, and that these areas will need to be addressed directly and explicitly in the course of therapy. The cognitive-behavioural approach to the treatment of bulimia has been worked out in detail, and has been more extensively researched than other approaches. Generally therapy will begin with an initial intense period of therapy, involving two sessions a week for one month. During this period therapy will focus on various behavioural techniques aimed at increasing control over the bingeing and purging behaviours. This will usually involve the client keeping detailed records of food eaten and methods of purging. Targets will be set that focus on establishing a regular pattern of eating which will tend to reduce episodes of overeating and food restriction. A range of 'stimulus control' methods will usually be employed as a way of helping the individual establish control over their eating behaviour. These methods focus on the sorts of conditions (or stimuli) that trigger the overeating response. Examples include: not engaging in other activities while eating; establishing set times and places for eating; limiting the amount of food that is available when eating; limiting exposure to foods likely to trigger overeating; careful planning of shopping lists and shopping; practice leaving food that is not required, etc. After this initial phase of therapy appointments may be reduced to once a week, and continue for between two and three months, making the total number of sessions up to 20. During this second phase a great deal of attention will be focused on identifying and changing dysfunctional, or problematic, thoughts. Much of this 'cognitive' work will address the distortions of thinking characteristic of the 'anorexic attitude', some of these distortions have been described in chapter 3 of this book. After therapy of between 12 and 20 sessions, several follow up appointments to monitor progress will usually be given, probably at intervals of three months. Similar approaches have been employed working with anorexics but have not been so extensively researched. The superiority of cognitive-behaviour therapy has not been established but it is one of the best researched approaches. Critics of this approach have argued that, as with psychodynamic therapy, the patient can easily experience an increased sense of ineffectiveness if the suggestions are not applied or fail to bear fruit.

The 'Existential' approach. 'Existential' is an inadequate term for what I have in mind, and many of those practising the approach would not welcome the label. However, there is a discrete, and important, body of opinion with a characteristic understanding of eating disorders and a particular approach to therapy which may loosely be described as existential. Counsellors or psychotherapists working from this position put great emphasis on the individual's experience of being anorexic or bulimic. As with psychodynamic psychotherapy, the existential approach to therapy involves taking the thoughts, feelings and fantasies, of the client very seriously and assisting her to understand the meaning of her symptoms. In particular symptoms will be seen as expressions of conflicts which centre on issues of identity, autonomy, sexuality and power. It is the individual's 'mode-of-being', of which symptoms are but an expression, that is the focus of therapy. Concerning this approach in the context of anorexia, psychotherapist Marilyn Lawrence and clinical psychologist Gill Edwards have noted: 'Since everyone is different, counselling sessions involve piecing together a different jigsaw puzzle for each person, of how they came to think and feel as they do about themselves, eating, body weight and life in general ... We feel that one can be most help by listening to someone who is anorexic; validating her feelings and experiences rather than telling her she feels that way because she is 'ill'; helping her to explore her present and past relationships; unravelling contradictions and false assumptions; and forming a trusting, one-to-one relationship as a basis for her personal growth ... Gradually, eating and body weight become less important, as the underlying problems are resolved.' This approach to therapy will not usually attempt to monitor weight or persuade the client to increase her food intake or monitor bingeing and purging with a view to reducing their frequency. These issues will be left to the client. Often a contract will be agreed that if a client's weight falls to a dangerously low level, therapy will stop and the client will be referred to her GP.

The above list is by no means exhaustive. But it does cover most of the therapies likely to be encountered in NHS settings.

As noted at the start of this chapter, research has not demonstrated the consistent superiority of any one form of therapy, and continuing diversity in theoretical orientation is likely to preserve distinct clinical approaches. This does make choice of therapy difficult. In practice what is available in a particular locality may impose severe limits on therapy options. Generally patients will be offered a combination of approaches, and individuals may well find some more suitable than others. The model of anorexia and bulimia as conditions with multiple determinants as outlined in chapter 3, suggests that various treatment strategies may be required to address the particular individual combination of causes which has led to the condition. Individual sufferers are bound to have personal preferences regarding therapy, hence it is important that the individual is offered an approach, or combination of approaches, that she feels she can work with and benefit from.

Outcome

Because bulimia was recognised relatively recently less information on intermediate and long-term outcome is available than for anorexia. But to summarise outcome research in a general way, it appears that at five years after onset between 70 and 75% of anorexics and bulimics will have recovered, or be significantly improved. Data from long-term follow-up of anorexics suggests that for between 20 and 30% outcome continues to be poor, although it has been found that the longer the follow-up the more people have recovered. It has been difficult to obtain mortality rates, but again it appears that the longer the follow-up the higher the mortality rate; so that studies indicate a 5 to 8% mortality rate four to eight years after onset, but in the long term (that is 20 to 30 years) this appears to be between 15 and 18%.

On choosing therapy and a therapist

Unfortunately not everyone will be in a position where they have a choice of therapy or therapists. However I strongly recommend making enquiries to see what is available locally. The Eating Disorders Association provides its members with an extensive list of local contacts which includes workers offering therapy in private and voluntary settings, as well as specialist and non-specialist NHS facilities. Membership of the Eating Disorders Association is currently £7.50. Your GP may also know of a range of contacts. Self-help groups are often invaluable as sources both of information about local services and of personal recommendation. If possible obtain personal recommendations from someone who has been in therapy for anorexia or bulimia and therefore has first-hand knowledge of a particular psychiatrist, therapist or counsellor. Whether you have a personal recommendation or not, it is important, especially if you are considering private therapy, to ascertain the therapist's credentials or training. Whether you are enquiring for yourself or your daughter, make sure you know what it is you are being offered; therapists will often want you to answer many of their questions, you have a right to expect them to answer a few of yours. Ask about their previous experience of working with people with eating disorders. It is also advisable to ask about the focus of therapy. As we have noted, anorexia and bulimia can be considered on two levels, one concerns the weight and food-related behaviours (e.g. food restriction, bingeing, purging, etc.) and the other concerns the underlying personal issues for which the eating disorder is both an expression and a way of coping. How does the therapist propose to approach these two levels? I would suggest that the focus should shift depending on the severity of the problem. When the condition is severe the priority will be to address the specific behaviours. Where the weight loss or the binge-purge cycle are less severe there can be a much greater emphasis on underlying problems. I am not suggesting there is a clear-cut line dividing the two approaches, but it is advisable to ask a therapist where the focus of therapy will be and under what conditions the focus will change. Sometimes the two approaches will be undertaken by different therapists, for example I have worked with anorexics where a GP monitored food intake and weight, and I focused entirely on the underlying difficulties. Whatever the arrangement, make sure you ask the therapist how he or she proposes to deal with emergencies, what are considered to be danger signs, etc. All these issues can be discussed at an initial consultation. Also, if you are considering a private therapist, make sure you are clear on fees, when they are paid, and the policy on missed sessions.

The process of therapy and recovery

Naturally the two most common questions asked by parents, concerned relatives and friends, are: 'Will she recover?' and 'How long will it take?' Both of these questions are always very difficult to answer. It was noted in chapter 5 that to a large extent both the success and length of therapy will be determined by two main factors: the duration and intensity of the condition prior to beginning therapy.

Hence, in general, someone who has been anorexic or bulimic for less than a year is likely to respond more readily to therapy than someone who has been anorexic or bulimic for several years. Also the greater the degree of weight loss, or the more frequently the bingeing and purging, the more difficult therapy is likely to be. As a general guide, where anorexia or bulimia has persisted for years, some form of therapy is likely to be necessary for between one and three years. However it must be emphasised that people respond to therapy in very different ways and some, it must be said, will not respond at all. As noted in chapter 5, people are likely to respond differently at different stages of the illness. During therapy the person with anorexia or bulimia gradually learns to deal with inner conflicts, feelings, and desires, in ways other than starving herself, or bingeing and purging. In order to genuinely relinquish anorexia or bulimia the person must have something to put in its place. This process of change naturally takes time, and is very unlikely to be a smooth sequence of improvement shown in terms of a continual reduction in symptoms. The process of therapy is usually uneven. Periods of improvement (measured in terms of reduction in symptoms) will often alternate with temporary increases in symptoms. If your daughter or partner is in therapy and you are alarmed by increases in symptoms, or perhaps changes in mood or behaviour that you find disturbing, contact her therapist or if this is not appropriate contact someone else involved in working with people with eating disorders, to talk about your concerns. It may well be the case that someone in therapy begins to express feelings when previously she would stay silent. There may, for example, be an increase in conflict as the anorexic or bulimic learns to express anger, resentments and disagreements. This process of change may be very wide-reaching and may come to embrace all of her relationships.

In conclusion, it is important to emphasise that while the majority of anorexics and bulimics who enter therapy make a good recovery, this does not occur without commitment and work on their part. No-one, and that includes therapists, can make a person move beyond anorexia or bulimia. Also families and friends should not assume they have a right to know what is said during therapy. The best approach is to ask her if she wants you to be involved and, if so, how? Having asked, respect her reply. There is no doubt that anorexia and bulimia are conditions that require effort and great courage to overcome. These qualities are needed not just by anorexics and bulimics but also by their families. Although living with anorexia or bulimia may be a great struggle, do not feel you are alone, avail yourself of the help and support that is available and the path to recovery will not seem so long.

Appendix 1
Useful addresses

THE EATING DISORDERS ASSOCIATION
Sackville Place, 44 Magdalen Street, Norwich, Norfolk NR3 1JE
Telephone helplines: 0603-621414 (Monday to Friday 9 a.m. to 4 p.m.)
0494-21431 (Monday to Friday 12 noon to 2 p.m.)

THE EATING DISORDERS ASSOCIATION
The Priory Centre, 11 Priory Road, High Wycombe, Bucks HP13 6SL
Telephone 0494 21431

EATING DISORDER ASSOCIATION GROUP
Dr Pat Hartley, Eating Disorders Department, Salford College of
Technology, Fredericks Road, Salford, Manchester
Telephone 061 736 6541 ext. 328 (office hours)

GREATER MANCHESTER COUNCIL FOR VOLUNTARY SERVICE
St Thomas Centre, Ardwick Green North, Manchester M12 6SZ
Telephone 061 273 7451 (office hours)

THE ANOREXIA AND BULIMIA NERVOSA ASSOCIATION
Haringey Women and Health Centre, Annexe C, Tottenham Town
Hall, Approach Road, London N15
Telephone helpline: 071-885-3936 (Wednesday 6 p.m. to 9 p.m.)

THE WOMEN'S THERAPY CENTRE
6 Manor Gardens, London, N7 6LA
Telephone: 071-263-6200

Appendix 2
Suggestions for further reading

Eating Disorders: Obesity, Anorexia Nervosa and the Person Within, Hilde Bruch (Routledge and Kegan Paul, London, 1974)

The Golden Cage: The Enigma of Anorexia Nervosa, Hilde Bruch (Open Books, London, 1978)

Anorexia Nervosa: Let Me Be, A. H. Crisp (Academic Press, London, 1980)

Anorexia Nervosa, Peter Dally and Joan Gomez (William Heinemann Medical Books, London, 1979)

Anorexia Nervosa and Bulimia: How to Help, Marilyn Duker and Roger Slade (Open University Press, Milton Keynes, 1988)

Anorexia Nervosa: The Broken Circle, Ann Erichsen (Faber and Faber, London, 1985)

Anorexia Nervosa: A Multidimensional Perspective, Paul Garfinkel and David Garner (Brunner/Mazel, New York, 1982)

Anorexia and Bulimia: Anatomy of a Social Epidemic, Richard Gordon (Basil Blackwell, Oxford, 1990)

The Anorexic Experience, Marilyn Lawrence (The Women's Press, London, 1989)

Fed Up and Hungry, Marilyn Lawrence, ed. (The Women's Press, London, 1987)

The Art of Starvation, Sheila Macleod (Virago Press, London, 1981)

Fat is a Feminist Issue, Susie Orbach (Hamlyn, London, 1979)

Hunger Strike, Susie Orbach (Hamlyn, London, 1986)

Anorexia Nervosa, R. L. Palmer (Penguin, London, 1980)

The Anorexia Nervosa Reference Book, Roger Slade (Harper & Row Ltd, London, 1984)